# Men Who Have Sex with Men

## Personality Attributes, PrEP, and Sexual Behavior

Personality Profile

Pre-exposure Prophylaxis (PrEP)

Sexual Behavior

Leonard I. Obodo

# Men Who Have Sex with Men

Research Findings

Abstract

Recent multicenter, randomized, double blind clinical trials have shown no association between HIV preexposure prophylaxis (PrEP) and increased sexual risk behavior among high-risk men who have sex with men (MSM). However, little research has been conducted under natural conditions devoid of clinical trial controlled environment to confirm the lack of association between PrEP and increased sexual risk behavior. Also, research has shown conflicting associations between sociodemographic characteristics and sexual risk behavior among MSM. In this cross-sectional, web-based, primary data analysis, MSM who reside in United States of America and who make use of PrEP for HIV prevention were examined to determine and explain the relationship between PrEP and sexual risk behavior using the theory of health belief model. In addition, the relationship between social demographic factors and sexual risk behavior among MSM was examined. The data were analyzed using logistic regression and the findings showed that the adoption of PrEP for HIV prevention did not significantly increase sexual risk behavior among PrEP users. The findings also demonstrated that all the social groups of MSM examined such as race, age, education, income, employment status, health access, and alcohol/drugs were not associated with risky sexual behavior. However, MSM who had full-time employment and those who were unable to work for health reasons were more likely to adopt PrEP for HIV prevention. The results from this study may help in the design of effective HIV prevention program for MSM and subsequently lead to healthy social interaction, respect, and friendship between MSM and the larger society.

<u>Men Who Have Sex with Men</u>

Personality Attributes

Pre-exposure Prophylaxis

Sexual Risk Behavior

# Dedication

This Book is dedicated to the memory of my late mother and father, Caroline and Theophilus Obodo, for their love, kindness, and mentorship that helped to shape my philosophy of life. Unfortunately, their early death left me with little or no opportunity to give back my love, warmth, and caring that they earned as hard working and loving parents. May their souls rest in the peace and love of the Almighty God.

Acknowledgement

My sincere and deep rooted appreciation goes to Dr. Rodney Lemery, for his

encouragement and advise during the difficult time of deciding on data collection method

for my research; and for his expert suggestions and insights that helped to improve the

quality of this book. I also thank Dr. Chester Jones for his contributions during the final

vetting of the various stages of my research. Finally, I am grateful to my family and

friends whose contributions may have directly or indirectly contributed to the quality and

standard of this book.

Table of Contents

iv

Chapter 1: Introduction

In 1981, five healthy men living in Los Angeles, California, were diagnosed with pneumocystis Carinii pneumonia (Chemicals et al., 2011). Two of the five men died of the disease which was later confirmed as Acquired Immune Deficiency Syndrome (AIDS) caused by Human Immune Deficiency Virus (HIV) (Chemicals et al., 2011). About 30 years after the discovery of HIV/AIDS, nearly 1.2 million Americans have died of the disease (Chemicals et al., 2011). Even though the introduction of highly active antiretroviral therapy (HAART) has been helpful in the reduction and stabilization of HIV/AIDS deaths, the number of new HIV infections remain high among men who have sex with men (MSM) and especially high among young men and those of minority ethnic groups (CDC, 2013a). The MSM who were infected with HIV/AIDS in the 1980s and 1990s experienced the devastating effect of the disease due to lack of full knowledge of the pathogenesis and therapeutic intervention needed to treat the disease (Chemicals et al., 2011). MSM and some support groups carried out a public campaign to draw the attention of the public health departments and the medical community to commit to extensive research and health policies; these led to the discovery of novel drugs for the treatment of the disease (Chemicals et al., 2011). Early sufferers of the disease therefore understood the need for safe sex and compliance with medical treatment.

Unfortunately, many young MSM who did not experience the epidemic and debilitating effect of HIV/AIDs seem to display complacency about its seriousness (CDC, 2013a). This is partly attributed to lack of knowledge of the cachectic images of full blown AIDS experienced in the 1990s in American communities (CDC, 2013a). The young MSM are therefore more likely to adopt inconsistent safe sex behavior and underestimate their personal risk (CDC, 2013a). They are also more likely to internalize

the false perception that HIV/AIDS is not a serious disease and more likely to be unaware

of their HIV status (CDC, 2013a).  These unhealthy assumptions have been shown to

increase risky behavior and increase the HIV infection rate (CDC, 2013a). The young

MSM are also more likely to be complacent about their partners HIV status because of

risky assumptions that drugs are available to make up for inconsistent healthy sexual

behavior (CDC, 2013a). Despite the complacency noted in younger MSM, healthy sexual

behavioral campaigns and programs delivered by many public health departments have

contributed to the reduction of HIV infections across many diverse groups (CDC, 2013a).

However, structural and sociodemographic impediments may be creating physical,

emotional and internalized apathy, which, in turn, may be contributing to increased risky

sexual behavior among MSM despite the healthy sexual behavioral programs (CDC,

2013a).

In order to reduce increased rate of new HIV infections among MSM, the CDC

has approved the use of daily preexposure prophylaxis (PrEP) to augment healthy sexual

behaviors among the men (CDC, 2013b). According to the CDC (2013b; Smith et al.,

2011), daily combined dose of tenofovir disoproxil fumarate (TDF) and emtricitabine

(FTC), called Truvada, was recommended for high-risk MSM and other high-risk

persons. The approval was based on results of randomized controlled trials conducted by

the CDC that showed 44-70% reduction in HIV infection among participants in the drug

arm of the study compared to placebo (CDC, 2013b; Smith et al., 2011).

While the need for a holistic approach to prevention the rising rate of new HIV

infections among MSM is acknowledged by the medical community, the potential barriers and the downside of PrEP (increased risky sexual behavior, drug resistance, long-term side effects, and informal use by people who are unaware of their HIV status) have not been fully studied (CDC, 2013b). Even though, the results of the Tenofovir/Emtricitabine (TDF/FTC) randomized controlled study did not show increased sexual risk behavior among research participants during the study period, real-life impact devoid of a controlled environment and risk counseling during clinical trials need to be studied for accurate assessment of the effect PrEP on sexual behavior. The findings from this study are expected to help to close this gap. Findings from this study are also expected to provide insights on the relationship between sociodemographic characteristics and risky sexual behavior among MSM; and how sexual behavioral changes compare among different demographic groups using PrEP for HIV prevention. Results from this study may introduce positive social change that may help improve healthy sexual relationships between MSM partners and couples; they may also help increase social interactions between MSM and other persons or group of persons with different sexual preferences and orientation.

Chapter 1 will therefore explain the following: background of this study, problem statement, purpose of this study and the research questions. Information on the nature of this study, the theoretical framework, and definition of terms; as well as the assumptions, scope, and delimitations are also provided. Insights on limitations, significance, and summary of the chapter is provided.

## Background

In 2010, investigators conducted a multinational randomized, double-blind clinical trial of daily prophylactic use of antiretroviral medications to prevent HIV infection among exposed and uninfected MSM (Smith et al., 2011). The result of the study and other follow up studies showed 44-70% reduction in HIV acquisition over a period of 6 months (CDC, 2013b; Smith et al., 2011). The investigators concluded that preexposure prophylaxis in combination with behavioral intervention may be needed to prevent rising HIV infection among high-risk MSM (Smith et al., 2011).

Based on the results of this clinical trial, the United States Public Health Service (PHS) Agency approved the PrEP regimen for MSM while more research is ongoing to determine the effectiveness of the use of preexposure prophylaxis for HIV prevention among MSM (Smith et al., 2011). The agency is concerned that the intervention program might lead to informal and unapproved use of HIV medications that have not passed clinical trials as well as the abandonment of safe sex practices or increased risky sexual behavior (Smith et al., 2011).  However, none of the clinical trials conducted so far have shown any evidence of increased risky behavior among MSM who participated in the trial (Molina et al., 2013). This could be explained by close risk counseling provided to the participants during the trial (Molina et al., 2013). Also, all the participants were either in the placebo or active (drug) arm of the study and may have been compelled to take extra precaution during the trial to avoid risky sexual behavior (Molina et al., 2013). While the medical community awaits the result of open-label studies of the use of PrEP among MSM, it becomes necessary to conduct a study to look at the behavior change from a real-life perspective devoid of health counseling and clinical research environmental modification (Molina et al., 2013).

A recent study in Australia showed that there is sporadic or informal use of HIV medication as prophylaxis by MSM; but the negative impact of such practice have not been fully researched (Zablotska et al., 2013). In this study, the relationship between PrEP and sexual behavior was examined in order to determine if the use of antiretroviral prophylaxis is associated with increased risky sexual behavior among MSM that may blunt the benefits of prophylactic use of antiretroviral drugs. Also, the role of social-demographic factors on sexual behavior was examined. Information from this study may help guide the PHS agency on the potential weaknesses or strength of antiretroviral prophylaxis among MSM. Also, findings from this study may provide insights on the demographic groups that stand the greatest risk of safe sex abandonment or relapse due to antiretroviral prophylaxis, so that such a group could be targeted for health education intervention and risk reduction counseling.

## Problem

In 2010, 63% of all new HIV infection in United States occurred among MSM; and 78% of all new HIV infections among all men in United States occurred among MSM (CDC, 2010; CDC, 2013c). Also, 72% of new HIV infection among young men aged 13-24 in United States occurred among young MSM (CDC, 2010; CDC, 2013c). Young African American men (aged 13-24) who have sex with men bear the greatest burden of new HIV infection in 2010, while Hispanic young men accounted for 22% of new HIV infection for the same age group (CDC, 2010).

Results from recent CDC analysis (2013d) demonstrated that MSM are disproportionately infected with HIV compared to heterosexual men in United States. Some researchers contend that reversing this trend will require an understanding of sociodemographic characteristics, perceived stigma, formal/informal use of HIV drugs as prophylaxis and risky sexual behavior among MSM (Kooyman, 2008; Zablotska et al., 2008; Francis & Mialon, 2010; Raymond, Chen, Stall, & McFarland, 2011).

According to Francis and Mialon (2010), MSM are discriminated against in work places, public places and social gatherings. The situation creates social, psychological and physical isolation of MSM from the rest of the community and this might have health consequences as these men may be compelled to engage in risky sexual behaviors (Francis & Mialon, 2010; Kooyman, 2008). Such risky behaviors may increase HIV infection among MSM (Semp & Madgeskind, 2000). It is also noted in the literature that some MSM have resorted to informal use of HIV medication before or after sexual encounter in order to protect against HIV infection. This emerging behavior may increase risky sexual behavior and the transmission of drug resistant HIV (Zablotska et al., 2013).

Supervie et al. (2010) provided insights on the use of mathematical model to predict the effect of Preexposure prophylactic (PrEP) intervention on HIV epidemic among MSM in San Francisco; they also highlighted how PrEP could reduce transmission of HIV infection while accelerating the transmission of resistant strain of the virus. It is feared that increased risky sexual behavior may be influenced by false sense of complete protection by PrEP regimen, with the possibility of increased transmission of resistant HIV (Supervie, García-Lerma, Heneine & Blower, 2010). So far, no quantitative study has been conducted to determine stable or increased risky sexual behavior with PrEP under natural conditions. Findings from this study may assist to close this gap.

In addition, poor adherence to the PrEP regimen may reduce efficacy and increase drug resistance (Bangsberg, Moss & Deeks, 2004).The issues of non-adherence to medication and the drug resistance of PrEP among MSM are influenced by the epidemic of multidrug resistant tuberculosis (TB) in New York City, where TB drug resistance was seen mostly in individuals who were non-adherent to medication as a result of addiction and mental illness (Bangsberg, Moss & Deeks, 2004). Lack of health care access may also limit procurement of tested, approved and recommended HIV regimen for PrEP (CDC, 2013e). People without access to health care may be motivated to seek alternative means of obtaining PrEP medication such as the Internet, with potential for the use of an unapproved and untested regimen with attendant drug resistance (CDC, 2013e).

The guidelines for the prescription of PrEP regimen by health care providers such as HIV screening at every renewal of prescription and other testing may encourage some individuals to look for an alternative, unapproved source of the PrEP regimen (CDC, 2013b). It is possible that the use of PrEP regimen by those who are already infected by HIV may accelerate transmission of resistant new HIV infection to a new partner which might lead to a futile cycle of resistant HIV epidemic (CDC, 2013b).

The relationship between age, public/family stigma, illicit drug, self-efficacy and risky sexual behavior among MSM have been extensively studied and found to be associated (Kooyman, 2008; Francis & Mialon, 2010; Raymond, Chen, Stall, & McFarland, 2011). While the existing literature is clear on the above psycho-social/demographic factors and risky sexual behavior, not much is known about the relationship between the use of antiretroviral prophylaxis among MSM and risky sexual behavior. In this quantitative cross-sectional study, the literature's lack of focus and clarity about the relationship between antiretroviral prophylaxis and risky sexual behavior among MSM and how this behavior varied across sociodemographic groups studied was addressed (Zablotska et al., 2013). Results from this study may be helpful in formulating effective and lasting preventive strategies that reduce the rate of risky sexual behavior among MSM (CDC, 2013c).

## Questions and Hypotheses

1.      Is the use of prophylactic antiretroviral medications associated with risky sexual behavior among MSM?

*Ho*1: Prophylactic antiretroviral medication is not associated with risky sexual behavior among MSM.

*Ha*1: Prophylactic antiretroviral medication is associated with risky sexual behavior among MSM.

Significance Level: Reject *Ho*1 if p-value < 0.05

2.      Do socio-economic status (SES), age, educational attainment, employment status, health care access, race and ethnicity predict use of PrEP among MSM?

*Ho*2: Socio-economic status (SES), age, educational attainment, employment status, health care access, race and ethnicity is not associated with use of PrEP medication among MSM.

*Ha*2: Socio-economic status (SES), age, educational attainment, employment status, health care access, race and ethnicity is associated with use of PrEP medication among MSM.

Significance Level: Reject *Ho*2 if p-value < 0.05

3.       Do socio-economic status (SES), age, educational attainment, employment status, health care access, illicit drug use, insertive or receptive anal dominant position, race and ethnicity predict risky sexual behavior among MSM?

*Ho*3: Socio-economic status (SES), age, educational attainment, employment status, health care access, illicit drug use, insertive or receptive anal dominant position, race and ethnicity is not associated with risky sexual behavior among MSM.

*Ha*3: Socio-economic status (SES), age, educational attainment, employment status, health care access, illicit drug use, insertive or receptive anal dominant position, race and ethnicity is associated with risky sexual behavior among MSM.

Significance Level: Reject *Ho*3 if p-value < 0.05

## Purpose

The purpose of this quantitative cross-sectional study was to determine the relationship between antiretroviral preexposure prophylaxis (PrEP) and sexual risk behavior among MSM who are currently using PrEP for the prevention of HIV infection in the United States of America (USA). Also, the relationship between sociodemographic characteristics and sexual risk behavior among MSM and how PrEP use varied across various groups of MSM was examined. In the first and third research questions stated above, the dependent variable is risky sexual behavior displayed by research participants during the period under research. Risky sexual behavior was defined as insertive or receptive anal sex without condom. The independent variables included: the use of PrEP, socioeconomic status (SES), age, educational attainment, employment status, health care access, illicit drug use, insertive or receptive anal dominant position, race and ethnicity.

Each independent variable was analyzed for potential association or no association with the dependent variable. The dependent variable for the second research question was formal/informal use of PrEP and the independent variables include SES, age, educational attainment, employment status, health care access, race, and ethnicity. Each independent variable was cross-analyzed with the dependent variable

Daily PrEP have been shown to reduce HIV infection by about 44-70% among study participants, but the role of PrEP under uncontrolled conditions have not been fully studied among MSM (CDC, 2013b; Smith et al., 2011). Results from this study may provide more insights on the role of PrEP and other structural and demographic factors on sexual behavior among MSM, as well as which demographic group may benefit more or less from its use for purposes of priority targeting and intervention.

### Theoretical Foundation

The theoretical framework for this study was the health belief model (HBM). The model provides insights about perceived benefits of action and barriers to action that help to explain people's participation in health-promoting behavior (Janz & Becker, 1984). The theoretical construct of the HBM consists of perceived seriousness, perceived susceptibility, perceived benefits, perceived barriers and self-efficacy (Janz & Becker, 1984). Modifiable variables such as demographic characteristics may influence the five components of the model, while cues to action (internal or external) may help trigger needed engagement in health-promoting behavior (Janz & Becker, 1984). The HBM provided needed explanation on the motivation for prophylactic use of antiretroviral medications by MSM and also provided insights on perceived barriers that may result in avoidance of safe sex behaviors while on prophylactic antiretroviral medication (Janz &

Becker, 1984). The modifiable variables and cues to action aspect of HBM helped to

explain how personal perception could be modified by certain variables and cues to

actions. This aspect of the HBM provided insights on the sociodemographic variables

such as level of education and how it could help inform the adoption of healthy life

behavior. Detailed explanations of various aspects of the HBM and how the model

related to this study approach and research questions are provided in chapter 2.

### Nature of the Study

This study is a quantitative, cross-sectional primary data analysis of the role of

preexposure prophylaxis and sociodemographic characteristics on sexual risk behavior

among MSM. The design is the best fit to answer the research questions and to analyze

both the exposure and outcome variables simultaneously (Bowden, 2011; Oleckno,

2002). Cross-sectional design was selected for this study because it is cost effective,

quicker and easier to arrive at results and conclusions. In this study, extensive description

of the relationship between the use of PrEP and sociodemographic factors and risky

sexual behavior among MSM was provided. Also, quantitative insights on the

relationship between sociodemographics characteristics and the adoption of prophylactic

use of HIV medications was addressed. The independent variables therefore included: use

of PrEP, SES, age, educational attainment, employment status, health care access, illicit

drug use, insertive or receptive anal dominant position, race, and ethnicity. The

dependent variables were risky sexual behavior and the adoption of PrEP by MSM.

Online data collection using web-based surveys was the data collection method for this study. MSM the living in the United States of America were selected as the population of study because the country has a large population of MSM who reside mostly in large cities such as New York and San Francisco (NYC Department of Health, 2011; San Francisco AIDS Foundation, 2011). Therefore, invitation to participate in the online survey required residency in the United States as an important inclusion criterion and was included in the online consent form. This helped to limit recruiting candidates outside the targeted population. A reputable online survey organization, with HIPAA compliance resources, was used to conduct the survey. Candidates were solicited by emails and social network websites frequented by MSM; they were given access to the survey website (Granello & Wheaton, 2004). Logistic regression was used to analyze the effect of individual predictor variable on the outcome variable. Also, logistic regression was applied to assess for effect modification of a combination of multiple predictor variables on the outcome variable (Oleckno, 2002; Green & Salkind, 2012).

## Definition of Terms

*Acquired Immune Deficiency Syndrome (AIDS):* AIDS is a disease that severely compromises the immune system of a person who is infected with HIV (CDC, 2012). The compromise of immune system involves inability of the immune system to fight mild infections and non-harmful bacteria that form part of the normal flora of the body systems, leading to opportunistic infections (CDC, 2012). The level of immune compromise in a person with AIDS is therefore determined by the CD4 cell counts and opportunistic infections (CDC, 2012). If HIV infection is untreated, the victim may die of AIDS in about 8-10 years from the time of initial HIV infection (CDC, 2012).

*Highly Active Anti-Retroviral Therapy (HAART):* Highly Active Anti-Retroviral

Therapy (HAART) is a combination of three or more HIV drugs used for the treatment of

persons infected with HIV in order to prevent the virus from becoming resistant to any of

the drugs (World Health Organization [WHO], 2014). Each drug in the combination

attacks the virus from different point in the synthetic pathway of the virus in order to

prevent the virus from multiplying in the system of the infected person (WHO, 2014a).

Therefore, HAARTS prevents the virus from attacking the victim's immune system and

makes the virus to remain quiescent and undetected in routine blood test, but remain

uncured in the victim's system (WHO, 2014a).

*Human Immunodeficiency Virus (HIV):* HIV is a virus contracted through the

exchange of body fluid from one person to another that could occur during sexual

encounter, breast feeding, blood transfusion, and sharing of unsterile needles/sharp

objects (CDC, 2014). The virus infects the immune cells of the victim and may destroy it

leading to inability to fight off infections. Over time, the infected individual may die of

AIDS (CDC, 2014).

*Modifiable Variable:* Modifiable variable are variables that could be changed by

certain actions or activities of the individual or the environment. Variables such as the

number of immunized and unimmunized children in a particular community could be

modified by the environment of the children such as the level of education of the parents

of the children in the community (Janz & Becker, 1984). High level of education may

lead to increased number of immunized children compared to the opposite (Janz &

Becker, 1984).

*Preexposure Prophylaxis (PrEP):* Preexposure prophylaxis (PrEP) is any medical action such as the use of medication, medical procedure and public health procedure administered to individuals or group of individuals before the exposure to disease causing entity such as HIV (Wade Taylor et al., 2013). In case of HIV infection, the PrEP is a HIV medication tested and approved for the prevention of HIV infection among high risk persons in order to prevent HIV infection among the group (Wade Taylor et al., 2013).

*Research Environment*: Research environment is the conditions that must be met at the beginning, during and after the research study that ensures valid results and conclusions from the research (Drezner & Golden, 2012). The research environment may include pre-treatment testing and counseling; regulated visit windows, maintenance treatment and testing. It may also include post-treatment testing or counseling and other regulated procedures (Drezner & Golden, 2012).

*Safe Sex:* Safe sex is when two sex partners agree and take adequate precaution to protect each other from sexually transmitted diseases and or HIV infection (Xiao et al., 2013). The precaution may involve the use of condoms or its equivalent by both partners among other precautionary steps (Xiao et al., 2013).

## Assumptions

In this study, it was assumed that participants to this web-based survey lived in the United States and provided honest answers to the survey questions. It is also assumed that study subjects knew the sociodemographic group they belong to and answered questions about this subject matter correctly and honestly. Also assumed was that all participants have knew healthy from unhealthy behavioral activities and the potential mode of transmission of HIV infection. It is possible that some people who are interested in participating in this study and who may be residing in other countries different from the targeted population may claim residency status of United States in order to meet the inclusion criteria for the study.

**Limitation**

This study was subject to several limitations. Online invitations to participants in this study may have been perceived by potential subjects as junk mails that may have been deleted (Wright, 2006; Konstan et al., 2005; Andrew, Nonnecke & Preece, 2003). Some of the invitations by Survey Monkey may have been mistakenly sent to the junk mails of the participants and may never have been red by intended participants (Wright, 2006; Konstan et al., 2005; Andrew, Nonnecke & Preece, 2003). The perception of the study invitation by the subjects as junk mail affected the sample size as many imminent participants may have declined the invitation. Many of the online audiences in this study were upscale, literate, upper-middle class persons with computers and Internet access (Wright, 2006; Konstan et al., 2005; Andrew, Nonnecke & Preece, 2003). They were also computer literate and had basic browsing skills with good online communication abilities (Wright, 2006; Konstan et al., 2005; Andrew, Nonnecke & Preece, 2003). These attributes may have helped to skew the target population to certain demographic groups and eliminated other demographic groups (Wright, 2006; Konstan et al., 2005; Andrew, Nonnecke & Preece, 2003). Lack of knowledge about how to navigate the online world and inability to express oneself in a computer may have turned off interested participants.

This, in turn, may also have contribute to the small sample size (Wright, 2006; Konstan et al., 2005; Andrew, Nonnecke & Preece, 2003).

Online surveys are problematic in achieving random sampling for a target population. Therefore, volunteers were used for this study and this may have affected the generalizability and internal validity of the results (Wright, 2006; Konstan et al., 2005; Andrew, Nonnecke & Preece, 2003). Some participants residing outside the targeted population may have been inadvertently invited and completed the survey. Some may have relocated to other cities or countries and may have received the invitation to complete the survey. Data collection from participants outside the targeted population were discarded and this may have affected the sample size as well as affected the internal and external validity of the result. Some participants may have declined to complete the survey for fear of revealing their personal information and other confidentiality issues. Others inadvertently provided personal information due to lack of computer and online communication skills (Bergeson, Gray, Ehrmantraut, Laibson, & Hays, 2013).

The issues related to using online surveys was minimized by using Survey Monkey and its custom audience targeting tools and skills to ensure that all groups in the population of study are adequately represented as well as increasing the sample size (Survey Monkey, 2014; Vives, Ferrecio, & Marshall, 2009). To avoid multiple entries by one participants, each participant was given access to one survey. The invitation to candidates explicitly stated the inclusion criteria for participation; the goal was to minimize the number of candidates who might have been disqualified. The invitation to participate provided all the measures taken to prevent breach of privacy and confidentiality such as deletion of IP addresses and personal information; these helped to reassure candidates privacy concerns (Vosbergen et al., 2014; Bergeson, Gray, Ehrmantraut, Laibson, & Hays, 2013).

## Scope and Delimitation

The scope and delimitations of this study consisted of participants who lived in United States; it excluded those who lived in other North American countries. Therefore, the results from this study cannot be generalized to the entire North American population. Also, this study did not take into consideration prior health education nor knowledge of the role of PrEP in the prevention of HIV infection. Finally, the cross-sectional design of this study did not allow for establishing causation between the exposure and outcome variables even when an association between the independent and dependent variables was significantly established.

## Significance

Risky sexual behavior is an important predictor of HIV infection among MSM (Osmond, Pollack, Paul, & Catania, 2007). This study was intended to demonstrate how one or a combination of sociodemographic factors predicts sexual behavior and HIV infection. Knowledge gained from this study could (a) assist in updating existing HIV preventive strategies and formulating new ones; (b) help to address the role of antiretroviral prophylaxis on sexual behavior among MSM that is currently under researched (Zablotska et al., 2013); (c) assist health care professionals to design cost effective and efficient programs that reduce risky sexual behavior among MSM, and to tailor a particular program to the demographic group that would benefit most. The combination of healthy sexual behavior and prophylactic use of antiretroviral medication may usher in an era of positive social change, manifested by healthy sexual relationships between spouses of MSM and partners, as well as healthy and favorable social interactions between MSM and the larger society.

**Summary**

Risky sexual behavior among MSM is an important predictor of HIV infection; a good understanding of personal activities and other structural and demographic factors are needed to design effective HIV preventive strategies for these men. The discovery and introduction of new pharmaceutical drugs as preexposure prophylaxis for HIV prevention needs to be adequately studied to determine how they impacts sexual behavior in order to avoid unhealthy sexual activities.

Therefore, chapter 1 provided an overview of why the role of sociodemographic factors on sexual behavior among MSM and the impact of the use of PrEP for HIV prevention needed to be well researched. The results and conclusions from this study may provide needed insights on how to design comprehensive, effective and cost effective HIV prevention programs and policies for MSM. The HBM was chosen for this study to explain the factors and motivation that predicts healthy and unhealthy sexual behavior among MSM. Chapter 2 will provide a detailed literature review, including the theoretical framework and a review of key variables, and a synthesis of literatures on the role of PrEP on sexual behavior.

Chapter 2: Literature Review

## Introduction

This chapter sought to provide insight into the research gaps related to the role of Preexposure prophylaxis (PrEP) and sociodemographic factors on sexual behavior among MSM. A healthy sexual behavioral program as a stand-alone strategy may not be enough to prevent the high rate of new HIV infections among high risk MSM in United States (Smith et al., 2011). MSM are currently disproportionately infected with HIV compared to other demographic groups in the country (Mith et al., 2011). Also, young and minority MSM aged 13-24 bear the greatest burden of the new HIV infection (Smith et al., 2011). According to CDC (2010), complementing healthy sexual behavior with PrEP have been shown to reduce HIV infection among high-risk MSM by about 40%. However, the impact of PrEP on sexual risk behavioral has not been adequately studied. Results from this study demonstrated the role and sexual behavioral implications of the introduction of PrEP to HIV preventive strategy among high-risk MSM. Also, results from this study might assist public health agencies to understand the contribution of social demographic factors on risky sexual behaviors that may contribute to high rate of HIV infections among MSM. The introduction of PrEP to high risk MSM may benefit certain demographic groups more or less. Therefore, the need to determine which group benefits most needs to be researched in order to maximize the effectiveness and efficiency of the PrEP strategy.

The literature review for this study consists of several major sections and each section provides an overview of how it contributes and/or complements other sections in providing insights on the research inquiry. The section on literature search strategy provided information regarding library databases and search engines accessed as well as key search terms and combination of search terms used to obtain the relevant literatures included or excluded in the research. The theoretical foundation is another major section in the review. This section describes major theoretical proposition for the theory selected for this study and why it was appropriate for the study. The theoretical foundation section also shows how the theory was applied in the past to explain similar research inquiry and how this study challenged or supported the application of the theory.

There were several major sections related to preexposure prophylaxis for the prevention of HIV infection among MSM. Some of the sections included the science of preexposure prophylaxis in the prevention of HIV infection among MSM, the PrEP strategy and barriers to PrEP. The sections provided details on existing literature on PrEP use for the prevention of HIV and how it is related to key variables of this study. Major sections of the literature review related to sociodemographic characteristics of MSM included the role of demographic factors on sexual behavior, the role of socio-economic characteristics on sexual behavior and the role of health care access on sexual behavior. Others included the role of race/ethnicity, nationality and substance use on sexual behavior among MSM. The literature on sociodemographic factors provided justifications for the choice of variables selected for this study and current knowledge and gaps discovered from the literature.

Finally, the literature review ends with an overview and summary of previous research methodologies and themes in the literature review and what is known as well as gaps discovered; and how this study fills one or more of the discovered gaps. The literature review concludes with transition and connection of the discovered gaps to the study methodology described in chapter 3.

## Literature Search Strategies

A careful search strategy, using Boolean operators and reputable library databases and search engines was conducted to locate articles for the literature review The following data bases and search engines were used: Medline, CINAHL Plus, PubMed, Google Scholar and the Cochrane databases. Also, the CDC public library and World Health Organization websites were searched for articles and other publication. The following types of literature were included: peer-reviewed articles, CDC research and policy publications, World Health Organization (WHO) publications and articles from *Mortality and Morbidity Weekly Report*. The key search terms and combination of search terms used for the literature search included the following: *Men and sex, Preexposure Prophylaxis (PrEP), HIV and MSM, PrEP and MSM and Truvada. Other search terms include: Age and MSM, Education and MSM, health care access and MSM and income and MSM. Also, Substance Abuse and MSM, Race and MSM and HIV* were other key search terms used. *New York City and MSM, San Francisco and MSM, Anal Sex and MSM, Insertive Anal Sex and MSM, Receptive Anal sex and MSM and Health Believe Model (HBM)* were also used during the literature search process.

The search conducted using theses search terms yielded 4,980 articles of which 180 relevant articles were selected and reviewed. Among these 180, 112 articles were excluded and 78 articles were included in the review. The inclusion criteria were as follows:

1.      Articles that are 10 years or less (2004 – 2014) except for articles/books on the foundation and fundamentals of research method and the Health Believe Model (HBM).

2.      Articles related to sexual behavior and HIV infection among MSM.

3.      Articles on the science of pre-exposure prophylaxis irrespective of the location of the study.

4.      Articles and publications on the fundamental principles of the HBM and its role in understanding and explaining HIV infections among MSM.

The exclusion criteria were as follows:

1.      Articles older than 10 years except those related to the foundation and fundamental principles of research method and the health belief model.

2.      Articles related to sexual behavior and HIV infection among females of any sexual orientation or preferences.

3.      Articles related to HIV transmission from mother to child.

**Theoretical Foundation**

**The Health Belief Model**

The HBM was the theoretical framework selected for this study. The Model was developed in the 1950s by three United States public health socio-psychologists named Hochbaum, Rosenstock and Kegel (Glanz, Rimer & Lewis, 2002).They developed the model to provide explanation and understanding about the failure of the public health tuberculosis screening program in the 1950s (Glanz, Rimer & Lewis, 2002). However, the model has been adapted to provide insights in the relationship between various behaviors and disease transmission especially on the relationship between risky sexual behavior and the transmission of HIV infection (Glanz, Rimer & Lewis, 2002). The model assumes that a person is motivated to take a health related action if the person feels that a harmful health situation could be prevented; and that taking recommended action could easily be accomplished.

The theory has been used to explain the adoption of sexual behaviors such as adoption of condom use, use of clean needles for drug injections and vaccinations for the prevention of human papilloma virus infection (Schneider et al., 2010; Reid & Aiken, 2011; Mehta, Sharma, & Lee, 2013). The potential behavioral changes related to the use of PrEP is similar to the adoption of condom use for the prevention HIV infection (Montanaro & Bryan, 2013). Therefore, the HBM was selected for this study because it helped to explain the motivation of behavior change in general while providing insights on sexual behavior risk for individuals on PrEP for HIV prevention; and the role of sociodemographic factors on sexual behavior (Schneider et al., 2010; Reid & Aiken, 2011; Mehta, Sharma, & Lee, 2013). The model consists of five elements which include: the perceptions of susceptibility, seriousness, benefit, barriers and self-efficacy (Janz & Becker, 1984).

**Perception of susceptibility.** Perception of susceptibility is when individuals perceive themselves to be susceptible to the risk of developing diseases and may be motivated to take preventive action based on the negative and severe consequences of the perceived risk (Janz & Becker, 1984). However, different people or group of people have different susceptibility perceptions. Some people have low susceptibility perception and may deny the existence of health risk and are more likely to engage in unhealthy behavior that increases risk of health issue (Mevissen, Ruiter, Meertens, & Schaalma, 2010; **Kilmer, Hunt, Lee, & Neighbors, 2007**).

On the other hand, some people have high risk perception and are more likely to adopt healthy behavior that reduces risk of disease (Janz, & Becker, 1984). **According to Leppin & Aro (2009) and Freimuth & Hovick (2012), sociodemographic characteristics and emotions may have indirect effect on perceived susceptibility to diseases.** Many public health preventive strategies strive to increase susceptibility perceptions of people by exploiting the strengths of susceptibility perception of health belief model in providing risk information to the public (Mevissen, Ruiter, Meertens, & Schaalma, 2010; **Kilmer, Hunt, Lee, & Neighbors, 2007**).

**Perception of Seriousness.** Perceived seriousness is the individual's subjective assessment of the seriousness of health issues (Daddario, 2007; Gerend, & Shepherd, 2012).The perception of serious harm to the individual by the disease entity or potential limitation of daily activities may lead the individual to engage in healthy behavior in order to prevent or reduce the severity of the health issue (Janz & Becker, 1984). People with high perception of seriousness are more likely to adopt healthy behavior compared to those with low seriousness perception (Janz & Becker, 1984) In addition to the individual's belief, perception of seriousness takes it root from familiarity with medical information and knowledge by the individual (Janz & Becker, 1984). A perception of seriousness from the same disease by different individuals could occur due to presence or lack of knowledge about the disease entity by different people (Asare, Sharma, Bernard, Rojas-Guyler, & Wang, 2013). It could also be due to demographic and geographic factors (Asare, Sharma, Bernard, Rojas-Guyler, & Wang, 2013).

Young MSM may perceive HIV as less serious and may be less inclined to adopt safe sex compared to older MSM or persons of different sexual preference. In similar situation, people in Africa perceive malaria as less serious disease and may be less likely to take preventive actions to avoid mosquito bites and malaria, while those in developed countries such as United Sates of America perceive malaria as very serious and are more likely to adopt healthy behavior to avoid mosquito bites and malaria (Asare, Sharma, Bernard, Rojas-Guyler, & Wang, 2013).

**Perceived Benefits and Barriers.** Perceived benefit is the individual's perceived usefulness of a new behavior in reducing or preventing the effects of a health issue based on the belief that the behavior is the right choice to achieve the desired health result (Janz & Becker, 1984). The adoption of the new behavior could be beneficial in primary prevention such as HIV prevention, eating healthy food to avoid heart attack; and secondary prevention such as screening for HIV in high risk group and early detection of breast cancer (Janz & Becker, 1984).

Perceived barriers are the individual's assessment of the obstacles that prevents the adoption of a new and healthy behavior (Janz & Becker, 1984). For an individual to adopt a healthy behavior, the obstacles to the adoption of the new behavior must be addressed (Janz & Becker, 1984). To overcome the barriers, the individual's evaluation of the benefits of the new behavior must outweigh the consequences of continuing the old behavior (Daddario, 2007; Gerend, & Shepherd, 2012). The barriers to the new behavior may include the opportunity cost of giving up the old behavior such as embarrassment, shame and personal discomfort (Janz & Becker, 1984). It may also include fears of adherence to the new behavior and accurate performance of the new behavior over a prolonged period of time (Janz & Becker, 1984).

**Self-Efficacy, Modifiable Variables and Cues to Action.** Self-efficacy is the belief in one's ability to perform or adopt a particular behavior based on the confidence entrusted in oneself (Janz, & Becker, 1984). Some individuals may evaluate a particular behavior as useful and healthy, but may lack the confidence to try and adopt the new behavior (Janz, & Becker, 1984). In this case, the perceived benefits of a behavior are negatively impacted by perceived barriers because of lack of confidence and self-efficacy (Daddario, 2007).

Personal perception in the health belief model could be modified by many variables and cues to actions. For example, sociodemographic variables such as education level, skills, past experiences among others (Janz & Becker, 1984). Persons who have been treated for severe influenza pneumonia and recovered are more likely to get immunized with influenza vaccine based on previous experience (Janz, & Becker, 1984).

Also, people who have been exposed to healthy behaviors based on their academic training such as nurses are more likely to adopt healthy behavior (Janz & Becker, 1984). Cues to action are activities that motivate people to adopt healthy behavior. Such activities include: media campaigns, personal acquaintances, advice from family members, friends and healthcare providers (Janz & Becker, 1984). The diagnosis of HIV infection in a close friend could be an important cue to action for a man to initiate screening for sexually transmitted diseases and other infectious diseases such as hepatitis B and C infections (Janz & Becker, 1984).

**Adaptation of HBM to PrEP and Sociodemographic Factors**

The potential behavioral changes related to the use of PrEP is similar to the adoption of condom use for the prevention HIV infection. Prior to this study, HBM has not been used to formally examine behavioral changes related to the use of preexposure prophylaxis among MSM (Schneider et al., 2010). Therefore, the HBM was selected for this study because it helped to build upon and expand existing knowledge of the motivation of behavior change; and also provides insights on sexual risk behavior for individuals on PrEP for HIV prevention and the role of each components of the HBM on sexual risk behavior (Schneider et al., 2010).

Previous application of HBM in research study show that key components of the HBM such as perceived severity and perceived vulnerability may not predict taking action to prevent infections such as encouraging condom use for the prevention of HIV infection (Hounton, Carabin & Henderson, 2005). Also, acquisition of health knowledge and knowledge of modes of transmission of infections may not translate to taking action to prevent infections. According to Hounton, Carabin & Henderson (2005), structural barriers such as poverty, gender inequality and other socio-cultural barriers was used to explain condom efficacy in a population of women at risk of HIV infection when knowledge of mode of infection transmission as well as perception of severity and vulnerability of infections failed to explain behavior change. Also, limited knowledge of the mode of transmission of disease entity may negatively impact on taking action to prevent diseases and may cloud the perception of seriousness and vulnerability. According to Jacobson (2011), high rate of HIV transmission among aging population (50 and above) in United States was partly explained using the lack of education and awareness of mode of transmission of HIV among the population. Applying the principles of HBM, a description of how the sociodemographic variables being tested pose positive or negative barriers to the adoption of healthy sexual behaviors among MSM similar to the findings of the condom use efficacy was provided.

## The Science of PrEP

The science of PrEP is based on the understanding and blocking of important steps in the life cycle and replicative process of HIV from the time and point of infection to final assembly of the replicated virus in the host body cells. Once infected, the virus attaches itself to the host immune cells in the organ of infection such as the sex organs, the mouth, rectum and similar organs of the body; and may also be transported to lymph organs of the host (Murray, Kelleher & Cooper, 2011). In the immune system of the host, the HIV attaches to the CD4 receptor cells and then deposits its genetic material into the host cells with the assistance of an enzyme called reverse transcriptase (Murray, Kelleher & Cooper, 2011). The reverse transcriptase converts the genetic material of the HIV to become similar to the host DNA so that the virus can enter the host cell with the help of another enzyme called integrase (Murray, Kelleher & Cooper, 2011). While inside the host cell, the HIV then uses the host enzymes to create long HIV proteins that will be used to create many copies of itself. As the virus creates long proteins in the host, it also starts the process of breaking the long protein into pieces of short protein using an enzyme called protease (Murray, Kelleher & Cooper, 2011). The pieces of the short viral protein can then be joined together with the viral genetic material to form new HIV virus. Therefore, the key target points in the replicative cycle include but not limited to the reverse transcription point and the protein synthesis point (Murray, Kelleher & Cooper, 2011). The science of drug intervention for HIV treatment and prophylaxis is based on blocking the reverse transcription replicative stage and the protein synthesis stage of HIV life cycle (Murray, Kelleher & Cooper, 2011). PrEP prophylaxis for the prevention of HIV is therefore based on blocking the reverse transcription step of the HIV synthesis (Garcia-Lerma et al., 2008). In this way, the virus will not be able to convert itself to simulate the host cell and cannot be integrated into the host genetic material and cannot multiply in the host cell. The host immune cells will then destroy the virus and filters it out of the host body system (Murray, Kelleher & Cooper, 2011).

Based on the pathophysiologic understanding of HIV life cycle, Subbarao et al (2006) examined the efficacy of tenofovir disoproxyl fumarate (TDF) chemoprophylaxis in the prevention of HIV in macaques and found that TDF protected against HIV in some and delayed HIV infection in others. However, the effect of TDF was not statistically significant which necessitated more research for combination chemo-prophylaxis. Further studies by Garcia-Lerma et al. (2008) examined the effect and efficacy of a combination of TDF and emtricitabine in the prevention of HIV in groups of macaques. Results from the study showed that the group of macaques treated with TDF-Emtricitabine combined PrEP have about 4-8 fold reduction in the risk of HIV infection compared to control group that did not receive TDF-Emtrictabine combined PrEP. These preclinical trials paved the way for the large scale phase III clinical trials in human populations at high risk for HIV infection which include but not limited to MSM. Also, Grant et al. (2010) and Molina et al. (2013) found that the combination of HIV medication (tenofovir disoproxyl fumarate and emtricitabine) as preexposure prophylaxis (PrEP) could be beneficial in preventing HIV infection in seronegative high-risk persons.

## The PrEP Strategy

In the last 20 years, the morbidity and mortality due to HIV infection as well as the rate of new HIV infection has declined across many demographic groups in the United States. However, individuals who engage in high-risk sexual behaviors and MSM have shown little or no decline in HIV infection rate (Kooyman, 2008). The PrEP approval in 2012 by Food and Drug Administration (FDA) as a preventive HIV strategy was based on compelling evidence of efficacy, cost effectiveness and lack of resistance and sexual risk behavior change for its use in HIV prevention among study participants (CDC, 2013f;Juusola, Brandeau, Owens & Bendavid, 2012). However, the efficacy rate was closely tied to the strict adherence to the daily supervised treatment protocol while lack of resistance to the treatment was linked to ensuring that all participants were HIV negative before the start of treatment regimen (Hurt, Eron, & Cohen, 2011). According to Marcus et al. (2013), there was no evidence of increased sexual risk behavior during the study period and immediately post study. Concerns for issues related to treatment adherence in the general population could pose some challenges in ensuring continued efficacy devoid of the emergence and transmission of resistant HIV strain in the population (De Man et al., 2013; Choopanya et al., 2013; WHO, 2012). Also, the strict sexual behavioral supervision and counseling during the PrEP clinical trials and the double blind design strategy that prevented the study participants from knowing which arm of the study (placebo or drug arm) they belong to could have prevented the study participants from engaging in risky sexual behavior throughout the study period (WHO, 2012). This raises concerns of replicating the findings of PrEP under normal conditions in the general public.

According to Paltiel et al. (2009), computer simulation modeled and adapted after the PrEP study show that despite increase efficacy in reducing the incidence of HIV infection, PrEP does not confer sufficient cost benefits to justify widespread use However, price reduction and easy access of PrEP especially among young and minority MSM would boost cost effectiveness and efficacy of the strategy. Therefore, potential facilitators to improved efficacy of PrEP and PrEP acceptability and motivation for adherence may involve free access to PrEP and other support services (Globus et al., 2013). Also, Bauemeister et al. (2014) found that young African American and Latino MSM are less likely to use PrEP if there is lack of free access to PrEP or if they lack health insurance to pay for it. Even as the cost barriers to adoption of PrEP and adherence to medication protocol remain a burning issue, internalized bias by physician prescribers of PrEP may affect equitable prescription of PrEP to all the demographic groups of MSM who may benefit from PrEP use. Calabrese et al. (2014) found that potential prescribers of PrEP perceive blacks as more likely than whites to engage in sexual risk behavior and therefore less likely to be prescribed PrEP medication for HIV prevention. However, there is no study or data on the sociodemographic variations in the current use of PrEP by MSM and this study intends to determine the factors that motivate different sociodemographic groups to adopt PrEP use.

These concerns may partly explain the conflicting efficacy results across large PrEP clinical trials conducted in many countries and across diverse demographic groups. The efficacy rate of PrEP clinical trials range from 44%-75% reduction in HIV infection to 49% non-significant increase in HIV rate in the Vaginal and Oral Intervention to Control the Epidemic (VOICE) trial conducted in women at high risk of infection with

HIV in Africa. So far, there has been one large phase III, randomized, placebo-controlled clinical trial (the iPrEx study) conducted across many countries spanning four continents among MSM and the result of the study show efficacy rate of 44% reduction in the incidence of HIV infection among the study population. However, the lower level of the 95% confidence interval was 15% as against 30% that is predictive of the need for public health intervention. These conflicting efficacy results underscores the need to conduct more research to determine how issues related to sexual risk behavior and drug adherence among MSM impacts on PrEP efficacy. Even though PrEP is not exclusively designed for only one high risk group (MSM), Tellalian, Maznavi, Bredeek & Hardy (2013) found that PrEP is prescribed more for MSM compared to other risky groups. Therefore, the study of PrEP use among MSM may provide better understanding of the strengths and limitations of the medication. This study selected MSM as target population to achieve better understanding of PrEP use and to help provide answers to many of the concerns discovered in previous PrEP studies.

Brooks et al. (2011) conducted mixed method study designed to determine potential adoption of PrEP and its impact on sexual risk behavior; and found that PrEP use might be associated with increased sexual risk behavior that may predispose to HIV infection. The result show that about 60% of study participants indicated that they may be compelled to adopt risky sexual behavior due to the perceived extra layer of protection from PrEP medication. The participants indicated likelihood to engage in anal sex without condom or use condom erratically and engage in sexual encounter with individuals who are HIV positive. This result is at variance with the findings in the large iPrEx study that showed lack of increased risk behavior among study participants. The methodology and design of the study was however based on future projections of intended adoption of PrEP use for the prevention of HIV infection that may not exactly translate to the behavior of individuals who are on PrEP medication for the prevention of HIV infection. This study intends to not only reconcile the conflicting results from these studies, but also to close the discovered gaps in the above studies by conducting the study among MSM who are on PrEP medication for the prevention of HIV infection and who are not subjected to stringent behavioral counseling and supervision.

### PrEP Barriers

Due to the stigma associated with HIV infection, the use of PrEP by HIV negative MSM may be falsely perceived by friends, family and community members as sign of definitive infection with HIV (Smit et al., 2012: Elst et al., 2013). Therefore, persons on PrEP may wrongfully be defined as persons living with HIV and may face discrimination from the community members unaware of the role of PrEP in the prevention of HIV. Elst et al. (2013) identified stigma related to persons on PrEP being perceived by community members as already infected with HIV and fears that such misconception could psychologically affect adherence to PrEP medication. The investigators also fear potential adherence issues and issues related to the refusal to adopt PrEP as HIV prevention strategy.

The interim guidance required for the prescription of PrEP regimen for HIV infection involves stringent prescription protocol (Norton, Larson, & Dearing, 2013). Some of the guideline includes documenting HIV negative status, confirming high risk behavior and establishing normal renal functions (CDC, 2011, January 28; Hosek, 2013).

Others include screening for hepatitis and sexually transmitted diseases; and providing risk reduction and medication compliance counseling (CDC, 2011, January 28; Norton, Larson, & Dearing, 2013). Also, 2-3 months follow up is required for renewal of prescription and establishing continued HIV negative status among other health related counseling (CDC, 2011, January 28). These stringent procedures and processes may discourage potential users of PrEP. According to Saberi et al. (2012), some high risk group of MSM may not be receptive to the use of PrEP based on concerns associated with these barriers; and Karris et al. (2013) suggested multifaceted programs that will help address potential barriers of real world use (other than clinical trial environment) of PrEP based on differing opinions and concerns of infectious disease physicians. This underscores the need to determine which demographic group will benefit most from PrEP and target such group for effective HIV prevention. This study sought to close this gap.

## The Role of Age on Sexual Behavior

The CDC data show that the rate of new HIV infection is rising among young MSM while the rate of new HIV infection among older MSM seem to have peaked. According to Balaji et al. (2013), the prevalence of HIV infection among MSM who are aged 20-22 years was higher than those aged 30 and above. Therefore, young MSM disproportionately bears the burden of persons living with HIV in United States compared to other demographic age groups. Also, Hampton et al. (2013) found that there is differential risk taking of young MSM across ethnic/racial lines. According to Hampton et al. (2013), older MSM aged 30 and above are more likely to report unprotected and risky sexual behavior compared to younger MSM and are also more likely to report HIV sero-conversion. Therefore, young MSM are more likely to be complacent in finding out their HIV status or the status of their sex partners. Also, young MSM are more likely to cover up their sexual orientation compared to older MSM and therefore more likely to engage in clandestine risky sex with unknown sex partners (Hampton et al., 2013). They are also less likely to be exposed to public health preventive program and other sex education programs designed to prevent sexually transmitted diseases including HIV infection (Hampton et al., 2013). It has been hypothesized that unprotected and risky sexual behavior among young MSM could be attributed to early onset of sexual activities before the age of 16 (Outlaw et al., 2011). At this age, young MSM are at increased risk of frequent sexual activity and more likely to use drugs; and also more likely to exchange sex for money (Outlaw et al., 2011). These sexual behaviors could vary according to ethnic/racial lines (Outlaw et al., 2011). In black families and communities, young age of men and being kicked out of the home for having sexual attractions or sex with another man is associated with risky sexual behavior (Warren et al., 2008). On the other hand, older age and ethnic identification among Latino MSM was associated with increased risky sexual behavior (Warren et al., 2008). For whites, no specific ethnic culture predictors have been associated with increased risky behaviors (Warren et al., 2008). However, Hampton et al. (2009) suggest inconsistency in the rate of HIV infection compared to the rate of risk taking across age groups among MSM. Hall, Byers, Ling, & Espinoza (2007) found that from 2000-2004, the rate of HIV infections within age groups did not significantly vary across ethnic and racial lines. This suggests that young MSM irrespective of racial/ethnic descent, may become vulnerable to the same psycho-social causative factors of risky sexual behavior. This study intends to reconcile the conflicting association of age and risky sexual behavior among MSM discovered in previous studies.

## Contribution of Race to Sexual Behavior

In United Sates, about 37% of all new HIV infection occur among Black MSM while 20% of the infection occur among Latino MSM (CDC, 2014b). Therefore, Black and Latino MSM are disproportionately infected with HIV (Calabrese et al., 2013). In 2009, 73% of HIV infection among all men occurred in black MSM (CDC, 2014b). The high rate of new HIV infection among Black MSM suggest that black MSM also disproportionately engage in risky and unhealthy sexual behavior compared to other group of men in United States (CDC, 2014b; Raymond & McCFarland, 2009). In this regard, black MSM are perceived by the general public as promiscuous, reckless and reservoir of HIV infection in the community (Raymond & McCFarland, 2009). Therefore, In MSM communities, blacks are least preferred as sexual partners and are more likely to be rejected in social venues where MSM socialize (Raymond & McCFarland, 2009). It is hypothesized that the discrimination compels black MSM to become interconnected among themselves with limited health information and HIV preventive services leading to acceleration of risky sexual behaviors and HIV infection (Raymond & McCFarland, 2009). However, there is no definitive consensus data to prove that risky sexual behaviors among Black MSM are peculiar and exclusive to them. Contrary to the hypothesized sexual promiscuity and reckless sexual behavior among Black MSM, Feldman (2010) and Millett et al (2012) found that black MSM lack some of the attributes that encourage risky sexual behavior such as increased number of lifetime partners, increased number of causal male partners and increased number of unprotected anal intercourse. As a result of conflicting data on rate of risky sexual behavior across racial lines among MSM, emphasis seem to focus on MSM network characteristics, structural factors such as education, incarceration, knowledge of HIV status and access to health care among other structural and upstream factors (Feldman, 2010; Millett et al., 2012). Also, structural factors such as issues related migration into United States and lack of access to health care and other social amenities may contribute more to risky sexual behavior among Latino MSM rather than differential risky sexual behavior compared across racial lines (Feldman, 2010; Millett et al., 2012). While it is reasonable to understand role of these structural factors on sexual behavior and HIV infection among MSM, it is also necessary to delineate the differential roles of risky sexual behavior across racial and ethnic lines and how it could help inform future preventive programs and policies.

### The Impact of Nationality on Sexual Behavior

The place of birth and the time of immigration into United States have been shown to be associated with risky sexual behavior among MSM (Oster et al., 2013; Brooks, Lee, Newman & Leibowitz, 2008). MSM who were born in other countries and who immigrated into United States and have lived in United for more than 5 years are more likely to engage in risky sexual behavior and be infected with HIV compared to those who have lived less than 5 years in United States (Oster et al., 2013; Brooks, Lee, Newman & Leibowitz, 2008). The high rate of HIV infection and risky sexual behavior among immigrant residents who have lived more than five years in United States are comparable to MSM who were born in United States (Oster et al., 2013; Brooks, Lee, Newman & Leibowitz, 2008 ). It is hypothesized that immigrant MSM may have faced hostile environment in their respective home countries and on arrival into United States were faced with a more favorable environment that encourages sexual freedom (Oster et al., 2013; Brooks, Lee, Newman & Leibowitz, 2008). Also, it is suggested that combination of lack of access to health care and other social amenities and perception of freedom of sexual expression could have predisposed immigrant Latinos who have resided 5 years or more in United States to risky sexual behavior and HIV infection (Oster et al., 2013; Brooks, Lee, Newman & Leibowitz, 2008).

## The Role of Educational Achievement on Sexual Behavior

The relationship between sexual risk behavior and level of education of MSM remain controversial, unresolved and inconsistent. According to Hampton et al. (2013) and Courtenary-Quirk et al. (2008), there is division among investigators in the link between higher education achievements and risky sexual behavior. Hampton et al. (2013) and Courtenary-Quirk et al. (2008) suggested association between higher educational and lower sexual risk behavior. Also, the investigators suggested a link between low education and high rate of HIV infection among black and Hispanic communities while acknowledging opposing findings. Therefore, research is needed to determine other factors that may act together or synergistically enhance the role of education on risky sexual behavior.

## The Impact of Income and Employment Status on Sexual Behavior

Individuals who are living with HIV infection and who have gainful employment and stable income are more likely to be mentally and psychologically stable and more likely to have better health outcome with the disease (Rueda et al., 2012). They are also more likely to have health care access and needed medication to fight the disease. According to Rueda et al. (2012), lack of employment or unstable employment as well as unstable income status is associated with poorer outcome among people living with HIV. However, it is unknown if income level, employment or stable employment status is associated with healthy behavior beyond the quality of life benefits provided by stable income and employment. This study intends to close this gap.

**The Contribution of Health Care Access to Sexual Behavior**

MSM have disproportionate access to health care facilities compared to other groups in United States (McKirnan, Du Bois, Alvy & Jones, 2013). Minimal or lack of access to health care could be attributed to lack of recognition of same sex marriage and the benefits that come with legal marriage such as health insurance for non-working spouse or partner (McKirnan, Du Bois, Alvy & Jones, 2013). The issues related to health care access among MSM may vary according to demographic groups and may negatively impact minority MSM more compared to other groups. McKirnan, Du Bois, Alvy & Jones (2013) found that demographic variations in health care access among MSM was related to lack of trust in the health care system, unwillingness to disclose sexual and other psychological constructs; and the perceptions of the surrounding health community as unfriendly. Therefore, some MSM may abstain from accessing the health care system for fear of encountering homophobic attitudes from health care personnel and for fear of disclosing their sexual orientation. It is also suggested that lack of health care access is associated with risky sexual behavior among MSM (McKirnan, Du Bois, Alvy & Jones,

2013). The missed opportunity of HIV prevention awareness, safe sex education and HIV testing that could have occurred when accessing the health care system may contribute to higher risky sexual behavior among MSM (Dorell et al., 2011). New York State and California have recognized same sex marriage and may be more receptive to MSM compared to other states. The impact of legalization of same sex marriage on health care access as well as perceived favorable attitudes towards MSM in these states need to be assessed and followed. This study intends to close this gap.

## The Impact of Alcohol and Illicit Drugs on Sexual behavior

Alcohol and illicit drugs are disproportionately consumed by MSM compared to other groups in the general population and has been suggested to contribute to higher sexual risk behavior compared to heterosexual men (Vosburgh, Mansergh, Sullivan, & Purcell, 2012; Dirks et al., 2012). Also, there is higher incidence of alcohol and illicit drug consumption in clubs frequented by MSM compared to clubs patronized by the general public (Vosburgh, Mansergh, Sullivan, & Purcell, 2012; Dirks et al., 2012). Cocaine and methamphetamine are the drugs mostly consumed by MSM and these drugs have been hypothesized to be associated with risky sexual behavior and increased HIV infection in the community (Vosburgh, Mansergh, Sullivan, & Purcell, 2012; Dirks et al., 2012). Also, stimulants and poppers were added to the list of illicit drugs independently associated with risky sexual behavior among MSM (Woolf-King et al., 2013). Heavy consumption of alcohol as a prelude to sexual encounter or during sexual encounter have been associated with increased sexual risk and HIV infection among MSM compared to heterosexual men (Vosburgh, Mansergh, Sullivan, & Purcell, 2012; Dirks et al., 2012).

Even though alcohol and illicit drugs have been linked to high rate of risky sexual behavior and HIV infection, not much is known about how alcohol and illicit drug impacts those who are on PrEP for HIV prevention. This study intends to close this gap.

## The Contribution of Anal Sex Position on HIV infection

Cultural behavior related to anal sex preference position has been shown to be associated with high prevalence of HIV infection among MSM (Zhou et al., 2013). Wei & Raymond (2011) and Zhou et al. (2013) showed that preferred anal sex positioning was an important predictor of HIV infection among MSM. Those who preferred receptive (bottom) anal dominant positioning were two times more likely to be infected with HIV compared to those who preferred insertive (top) dominant position. Also, the preference for bottom position varied across demographic groups, with low educated men and men from Asian/Pacific Islanders preferring bottom position compared to other racial and level of education categories (Wei & Raymong, 2011). However, the authors did not look at other demographic characteristics such as age and how it predicts anal sex position preference and HIV infection rate. Since the rate of new HIV infection is higher among young MSM, it is important to examine all potential demographic characteristics that predict new HIV infection in young MSM. This study intends to close this gap.

## Overview of Methodologies and Literature Gaps

The synthesis of past research methodology related to this study revealed that most of the investigators deployed the use of cross-sectional research method which is the method selected for this study. However, the initial multinational and multicenter

PrEP study was basically a phase III randomized, controlled, double blind clinical trial to determine the efficacy of PrEP for the prevention of HIV infection and sexual risk compensation among high risk groups. According to Marcus et al. (2013), there was no evidence of increased sexual risk behavior among study participants in the PrEP clinical trial. This conclusion was arrived at by comparing baseline interview-administered questionnaire with post trial questionnaire completed by the study participants (Marcus et al., 2013). However, the study participants were blinded to active and placebo arm of the study and could possibly abstain from sexual risk behavior during the study window. Also, instructions and counseling during study period may have inadvertently enlightened the participants on the need to adopt safe sex throughout the duration of the study; and that may have affected sexual behavior risk among the participants. Conclusions from the PrEP clinical trial exposed innovative HIV preventive opportunities while revealing challenging weaknesses that need further inquiry. The challenging weaknesses of the PrEP clinical trial triggered many follow up studies with cross-sectional design to further provide insights on the potential issues related to increased sexual behavior risk among HIV high risk group.

Therefore, this study was conducted because of the need to determine the influence of PrEP on increased sexual behavior risk under uncontrolled and un-blinded condition that is close to natural situation in order to help provide more clarity to the influence of PrEP on sexual behavior. Similarly, Brookes et al. (2012) conducted a cross-sectional study to determine potential adoption of a hypothetical PrEP for HIV prevention and potential sexual behavior change associated with PrEP use. Results of the study show that 64% of the participants indicated potential likelihood to adopt risky sexual behavior due to potential perception of safety from the medication while 60% of the participants indicated likelihood to abandon condom use (Brookes et al., 2012). This finding seem to contradict the PrEP clinical trial finding. Similar hypothetical cross-sectional study conducted by Golub et al. (2012) show that 68.5% of the study participants reported likelihood to adopt PrEP use for HIV infection but also indicated 35% likelihood to decrease or abandon condom use while on PrEP. Demographic breakdown also show that participants who indicated likelihood to abandon condom use were more likely to have college degree and belong to high income bracket (Golub et al., 2012). However, there was no difference in sexual risk behavior across racial groups. Issues related to ambiguity, ambivalence and apprehension of the use of PrEP for HIV infection and potential increased behavior risk was studied by Saberi et al. (2012) using cross-sectional study method. The investigators found that individuals of greatest risk for HIV infection were less likely to adopt PrEP while those of moderate risk indicated more interest in PrEP but also indicated likelihood for increased sexual risk behavior while on PrEP. Even though studies conducted by Brookes et al (2012), Golobs et al. (2013) and Saberi et al. (2012) contradicted the PrEP clinical trial finding, the studies were hypothetical and was conducted among MSM who were not actively on PrEP medication. I intend to close the research methodology gaps discovered and the conflicting results from previous research.

Synthesis of past study methods regarding the role of sociodemographic characteristics and sexual risk behavior were conducted using cross-sectional research method which is also the method adopted for this study. Hampton et al. (2013) conducted a study to determine the relationship between age, education and sexual risk taking among African American MSM residing in New York City (NYC). Results from the study show that sexual risk behavior were more likely to be reported by participants with low educational achievements while race and age were not significantly associated with sexual risk behavior. In similar cross-sectional study conducted to determine the relationship between health care access and sexual behavior among MSM, McKirnan et al. (2013) found that 27% of the participants reported 0 or 1 health care access indicator. The investigator also found that black and Latino race as well as low income people were mostly impacted with limited access to health care. Also, overall lack of health care access was associated with risky sexual behavior. Warren et al. (2008) conducted a cross-sectional study to determine the predictive factors of unprotected sex among MSM in Chicago, Miami-Dade and Broward County, Florida and found that younger age of initiation of sex was associated with increased sexual risk behavior among African American youths while ethnic identification and older age were associated with increased sexual risk behavior among Latino MSM. On the other hand, there was no known ethnic/racially related predictors associated with increased sexual risk among white youths. In the light of above contradictory findings in previous studies, more studies are needed to determine the relationship between individual sociodemographic factor as well as combination of the factors and sexual risk behavior. This study intends to examine many sociodemographic and structural factors in one cross-sectional study design in order to help close the conflicting research findings and conclusions from previous studies.

## Summary and Conclusion

Four decades after HIV epidemic and HIV intervention with highly active anti-retroviral therapy (HAART) in United States, the number of new HIV infection remain high among MSM and especially high among young men of minority ethnic descent (CDC, 2010a; CDC, 2013c). According to the CDC (2010a; 2013c), current public health education on safe sex and other risky behavior modification may not be enough to reduce the rising rate if HIV among MSM. To this regards, the approval and introduction of PrEP may help reduce the rising rate of HIV infection among MSM (Smith et al., 2011). However, the implications of PrEP on increased sexual risk behavior has not been fully researched. In addition, the differential adoption of PrEP for the prevention of HIV infection has not been fully studies across different sociodemographic groups in order to determine the most likely group to benefit most from PrEP program. Even though personal behavioral risk factors are important predictor of HIV infection, more research is also needed to determine the role of different structural and sociodemographic factors in the enhancement of HIV infection among MSM. Currently, there is much contradictory data on the role of different types of social, economic and demographic factors on sexual risk behavior and HIV infection. Public health scholar practitioners agree that a holistic preventive approach is needed to prevent resurgence of HIV epidemic among MSM (Smith et al., 2011). In this study, the natural role of PrEP program on sexual risk behavior different from the artificial environment created during previous studies on the role of PrEP on sexual risk behavior was examined. Since individual behavioral risk is an important predictor of HIV infection, good knowledge of the role of PrEP on sexual risk behavior may help public health program designers and policy makers to develop guidelines for PrEP use and then tailor them to the demographic groups who will benefit most. Chapter 3 will describe detailed aspects of this research method which include but not limited to the study design, population of study, sampling strategy, measurement tools, data collection, threat to internal validity and data analysis.

Chapter 3: Research Method

**Introduction**

The purpose of this quantitative cross-sectional study is to determine the relationship between the use of preexposure prophylaxis (PrEP) and sexual risk behavior among MSM residing in the United States. In addition, the relationship between sociodemographic factors and sexual risk behavior was quantitatively examined. The need to re-examine the relationship between PrEP and sexual risk behavior was based on concerns and gaps in the design and methodology of the PrEP clinical trials. Results from the multicenter, multinational, randomized, controlled clinical trials showed that daily dose of preexposure prophylaxis (PrEP) reduced HIV infection by 44-70% among high risk men who have sex with men (MSM) (CDC, 2013b; Smith et al., 2011). The result from the clinical trial also showed that there was no evidence of increased sexual risk behavior among the study participants throughout the duration of the clinical trial (CDC, 2013b; Smith et al., 2011). However, there is a concern that the results from the PrEP clinical trial may not reflect the real-life sexual risk behaviors of the participants (that is, in the absence of the controlled environment in a clinical trial). Thus, the results from this study revealed more insights on the role of PrEP and other structural and demographic factors on sexual behavior among MSM along with demographic group may benefit more or less from its use (for purposes of priority targeting and intervention).

Chapter 3 provides the following details: the research design for this study and the rationale for its selection as well as concise explanation of the dependent and independent variables; comprehensive information on sampling procedures, sample size calculation and procedures for recruiting subjects; explanation of the threats to validity and reliability of the measurement instrument as well as data collection procedures; the plan to address any ethical concerns related to anonymity of the participants and confidentiality of the data collection materials.

## Research Design and Rationale

This study was a quantitative, cross-sectional primary data analysis of the role of Sociodemographic characteristics and antiretroviral prophylaxis on sexual risk behavior among men who have sex with men (MSM) (Oleckno, 2002). The design was chosen because it was expected to help expose patterns that might suggest an association between predictors of health conditions and health outcomes and that this might help inform strategies for future studies. In addition, the cross-sectional design was selected for this study because it is a good fit for investigating the relationship between one or multiple risk factors and the outcome of interest simultaneously for purposes of understanding a disease process and for public health planning (Oleckno, 2002). Using aa cross-sectional design and a web-based survey is inexpensive, less time consuming and less cumbersome compared to other research designs to arrive at study results and conclusions (Oleckno, 2002). The result from this study may help provide insights into planning public health HIV prevention programs for MSM. Conclusion from this study may also provide more insights into the formulation of hypothesis that would support further studies to advance and update current knowledge in HIV prevention among high-risk MSM.

## Research Questions, Hypotheses and Variables

Research Question 1 (RQ1): Is use of prophylactic antiretroviral medications associated with risky sexual behavior among MSM?

*Ho*1: Prophylactic antiretroviral medication is not associated with risky sexual behavior among MSM.

*Ha*1: Prophylactic antiretroviral medication is associated with risky sexual behavior among MSM.

Significance Level: Reject *Ho*1 if p-value < 0.05

Dependent Variable: The dependent variable in research question #1 is the sexual risk behavior of the research participants. Sexual risk behavior is a categorical variable represented on nominal scale and captured in likert format (Yes/No) (Frankfort-Nachmias & Nachmias, 2008).

Independent Variable: The independent variable in research question #1 is the use of preexposure prophylaxis (PrEP) by the research participants. PrEP use is a categorical variable represented on nominal scale and captured in Likert format (Yes/No) (Frankfort-Nachmias & Nachmias, 2008). The independent variables (PrEP) were cross-tabulated with the dependent variable (Sexual risk behavior) and statistically analyzed using binary logistic regression.

Research Question 2 (RQ2): Do socio-economic status (SES), age, educational attainment, employment status, health care access, race and ethnicity predict use of PrEP among MSM?

*Ho*2*:* Socio-economic status (SES), age, educational attainment, employment status, health care access, race and ethnicity is not associated with use of PrEP medication among MSM.

*Ha*2: Socio-economic status (SES), age, educational attainment, employment status, health care access, race and ethnicity is associated with use of PrEP medication among MSM.

Significance Level: Reject *Ho*2 if p-value < 0.05

Dependent Variable: The dependent variable in research question #2 is the use of preexposure prophylaxis (PrEP) by research participants and the characteristics of the variable as described in research RQ1 also applies.

Independent Variables: The independent variables in question #2 are age, educational attainment, employment status, health care access, race/ethnicity and socio-economic status. Age of participants is a categorical variable represented in nominal scale and divided into three groups (18-30, 31-64, 65 and above) (CDC, 2010b; Frankfort-Nachmias & Nachmias, 2008). Race of participants is a categorical variable represented in nominal scale and divided into six groups-White, Black, Hispanic, American Indian, Asian and Native Hawaiian (CDC, 2010b; Frankfort-Nachmias & Nachmias, 2008). Employment status of participants is a categorical variable represented in nominal scale and divided into seven groups (employed full time, employed part-time, a home maker, full time student, retired, unable to work due to health reasons, unemployed) (CDC, 2010b; Frankfort-Nachmias & Nachmias, 2008). Health care access of participants is a categorical variable represented in nominal scale and divided into two groups (access to health and no access to health care) (Frankfort-Nachmias & Nachmias, 2008).

Educational attainment of participants is a categorical variable represented in nominal

scale and divided into seven groups (never attended school, Grade 1-8, Grade 9-11,

Grade 12 or GED, some college degree, bachelor's degree, some post graduate

education) (CDC, 2010b; Frankfort-Nachmias & Nachmias, 2008). Income level of

participants is a categorical variable represented in nominal scale and divided into

thirteen groups (CDC, 2010b; Frankfort-Nachmias & Nachmias, 2008). Each

independent variable stated above was cross-tabulated with the dependent variable (use

of PrEP) and statistically analyzed using binary logistic regression.

Research Question 3 (RQ3): Do socio-economic status (SES), age, race/ethnicity,

educational attainment, employment status, health care access, illicit drug use, insertive

or receptive anal dominant position, race and ethnicity predict risky sexual behavior

among MSM?

*H*o3): Socio-economic status (SES), age, educational attainment, employment

status, health care access, illicit drug use, insertive or receptive anal dominant position,

race and ethnicity is not associated with risky sexual behavior among MSM.

*H*a3: Socio-economic status (SES), age, educational attainment, employment

status, health care access, illicit drug use, insertive or receptive anal dominant position,

race and ethnicity is associated with risky sexual behavior among MSM.

Significance Level: Reject *H*o3 if p-value < 0.05

Dependent Variable: The dependent variable in RQ3 is the use of preexposure prophylaxis (PrEP) by research participants and the characteristics of the variable as described in RQ1 also applies.

Independent Variable: The independent variable in research question #3 are socio-economic status (SES), age, race/ethnicity, educational attainment, employment status, health care access, illicit drug/alcohol use, insertive or receptive anal dominant position, and race/ethnicity. Insertive or receptive anal dominant position preference of participants is a categorical variable represented in nominal scale and captured in Likert format (Yes/No) (CDC, 2010b; Frankfort-Nachmias & Nachmias, 2008). Illicit drug/alcohol use of participants is a categorical variable represented in nominal scale and divided into three groups (drug use, alcohol use and simultaneous drug and alcohol use) (CDC, 2010b; Frankfort-Nachmias & Nachmias, 2008). Other independent variables are similar to the independent variables narrated in RQ2. Each independent variable stated above was cross-tabulated with the dependent variable (sexual risk behavior) and statistically analyzed using binary logistic regression.

**Target Population**

MSM residing in United States were the study population for this study. United States was selected as the population of study because the country has a large population of MSM especially in major cities such as New York and San Francisco among other cities (NYC Department of Health, 2011; San Francisco AIDS Foundation, 2011). For example, most of the MSM in New York State (272,493) reside in New York City (Gates, 2006). Most MSM in California State reside in San Francisco, San Diego and Sacramento with population of 94, 234; 61,945; and 32,108 respectively (Gates, 2006).

The invitation to participate in the online survey required residency in USA as an important inclusion criterion and was included in the online consent form. This helped to limit recruiting respondents outside the targeted population.

### Sampling and Sampling Procedures

An unrestricted self-selected web-based survey was the sampling method selected for this study. It is a type of non-probability (convenience) sampling that allows any interested member of the targeted population to participate in the web-based survey (Greenlaw & Brown-Welty, 2009). Convenience sampling was selected for this study because the targeted population is difficult to reach; and the sampling method is comparatively inexpensive, involves minimal efforts and requires less time to accomplish result (Greenlaw & Brown-Welty, 2009). All interested MSM residing in United States who signed the informed consent form and who is 18 years and above was included in the study. On the other hand, all MSM who did not sign the informed consent and who is residing in countries and places outside the United States were excluded from the study. Heterosexual men and homosexual females were also excluded from the study.

### Sample Size Calculation

The sample size of 73 participants was calculated using prevalence rate of risky sexual behavior among MSM, confidence level of 95% and margin of error of 5% (University of North Carolina, 2010). Based on recent research, the prevalence rate of risky sexual behavior among MSM is 2.5% (Rosenberger et al., 2012). Confidence level of 95% was selected because 95% of the sample are expected to contain the true population parameter and alpha level of 0.05 was selected in order to optimize the sample size for this study (UNC, 2010). In this study, it was assumed that the prevalence rate of risky sexual behavior among MSM is 5% (two times the estimated prevalence rate) in order to increase sample size for the study.

**Sample Size Formula**

$n = T^2 \times P(1-P) / ME^2$

$n$ = sample size

$T$ = confidence level at 95% (1.96)

$P$ = estimated prevalence (5% or 0.05)

$ME$ = margin of error at 5% (0.05)

$n = (1.96)^2 \times 0.05 (1 - 0.05) / (0.05)^2$

$n = 3.8416 \times 0.05 \times 0.95 / 0.0025$

$n = 0.182476 / 0.0025$

$n = 73$

## Recruitment and Data Collection Procedures

Survey Monkey website was used to create the web-based survey for this research which lasted for three months. Survey Monkey is a reputable online survey organization with HIPAA compliant resources that allows users (individuals, academic institutions and cooperate organizations) to create web-based surveys and collect responses from various users of the internet. Survey questions and online consent tool were delivered to the participants through custom web-link created for this study. Participants were solicited by emails and social network websites frequented by MSM. Also, Survey Monkey Organization sent out emails to custom audience of MSM to solicit for participants. In addition, business cards with survey website was distributed to local bars and bathhouses patronized by MSM. Access to the survey page was provided to interested participants who had consented to participate in the survey. Social network organizations and clubs that provide social services and recreational activities for MSM helped to disseminate and advertise information about the study by making the survey link accessible to interested participants. Interested participants were requested to click on the survey link or copy and paste the link to their web browser to access the informed consent page. The participants were requested to read the electronic informed consent form and then agree or disagree to participate by clicking the next button or by closing the web-page and exiting the survey page respectively. Detailed content of the electronic consent form is provided in the appendix section. By clicking the next button, the survey questionnaire was activated for the participants to complete the survey questions. The active survey questionnaire was divided into four sections which include: demographic characteristics, sexual behavior, HIV testing and HIV preexposure prophylaxis (CDC, 2010b). The demographic characteristics collected include: age, ethnicity, sexual orientation, marital status and country of birth. Others include level of education, employment status, income level, housing condition and health care access. Details of the questions on various sections of the questionnaire is provided in the appendix section. Participants were free to skip any question and could also move back and forth the pages of the active survey questions as they wish. The next button was located in the last page of the survey and participants were directed to return to previous page or to click the submit button to submit the survey. Each participant could access the survey questions several times by saving the answers to return at a later time. However, once the survey was submitted, the participants were unable to access the survey questions to make further changes and were thanked for participating in the survey. There was no follow up or debriefing procedures for this study. The results of the survey was delivered in word, PDF, and SPSS document by Survey Monkey with secured password.

## Instrumentation

The National HIV Behavioral Surveillance System (NHBSS) questionnaire was the data collection instrument selected for this study. The instrument was developed in 2003 by the CDC in conjunction with 25 states and local public health departments in United States (MacKellar et al., 2007). It is one of the most valid and reliable tools for monitoring HIV risk behavior in United States (MacKellar et al., 2007). The instrument was developed to target HIV high risk population which include men who have sex with men, injecting drug users and high risk heterosexual individuals (MacKellar et al., 2007). Also, the purpose of the tool was to determine behaviors that help to accelerate HIV infection among the high risk groups so that HIV prevention strategic plan could be developed to monitor the high risk behavior and HIV epidemic among the groups (MacKellar et al., 2007). The tool was designed to collect cross-sectional data on HIV behavior risk factors which is the format selected for this study and which makes it appropriate data collection tool for this study. Permission to use the NHBSS questionnaire for this study was not obtained because the data collection tool was produced by a federal agency and displayed in public domain and can be reproduced without permission as long as published articles derived from the tool acknowledges the federal agency (CDC, 2013g). Some of the data collected using the NHBSS questionnaire included demographic characteristics, sexual behavior, drug use, HIV testing, health care access, and preexposure prophylaxis (MacKellar et al., 2007). The practical interpretation and use of the NHBSS data was based on the proportion of at risk persons who had unprotected sex or multiple sex partners in the previous 12 months as well as those who injected/shared needles in the last 12 months (MacKellar et al., 2007). The validity of the tool have been shown to be consistent over many years and in different settings and groups; and generalizability may be drawn from studies that made use of the tool depending on the study design (MacKellar et al., 2007). The limitation of the NHBSS instrument is that it could be subject to social desirability biases due to the self-report nature of the instrument (MacKellar et al., 2007). However, this bias was minimized by the anonymous nature and confidentiality safeguards incorporated into the tool (MacKellar et al., 2007).

## Data Analysis Plan

Statistical Package for the Social Science (SPSS) was the statistical software selected to analyze the data collected for this study. SPSS was selected because the tool is fast in analyzing data and also has inbuilt techniques for data cleaning (Green & Salkind, 2012). The software also has variety of statistical methods and graphs available to investigators and stores output results in separate files. Prior to SPSS analysis of the data collected during this study, data screening and cleaning of the raw survey data was performed manually and electronically using the various techniques available in the SPSS software. Data screening and cleaning is the process of identifying and rectifying potential errors in survey data before performing final statistical analysis of the data collected. The survey raw data was checked manually for the eligibility of participants to ensure that the participants met the inclusion criteria which include signing of the informed consent forms, eligibility age and place of residence. Also, personal identifiers such as IP addresses, names, and home addresses of participants was deleted if inadvertently provided and not automatically deleted by Survey Monkey software. At the end of initial manual data screening and cleaning, data was entered into the SPSS tool in preparation for data analysis. The SPSS tool was deployed to perform final data cleaning using the frequency technique to detect transcription errors that may have occurred during data entry into the SPSS.

**Hypothesis 1**

*Ho*1: Prophylactic antiretroviral medication is not associated with risky sexual behavior among MSM.

*Ha*1: Prophylactic antiretroviral medication is associated with risky sexual behavior among MSM.

The independent variable from above hypothesis is the use of preexposure prophylaxis and the dependent variable is risky sexual behavior of the participant. Descriptive statistics was conducted to generate frequency distribution table for the independent variable to show the frequencies and percentages of those who use and who do not use preexposure prophylaxis. The values of the independent variable was cross-tabulated with the values of the dependent variable and binary logistic regression was conducted to determine the association between the two. The concept of odds ratio (EXP

(B), the Sig (p-value) and 95% confidence internal (95% CI) was used to interpret the presence or absent of an association between the dependent and independent variable.

**Hypothesis 2**

*Ho*2: Socio-economic status (SES), age, educational attainment, employment status, health care access, race and ethnicity is not associated with use of PrEP medication among MSM.

*Ha*1: Socio-economic status (SES), age, educational attainment, employment status, health care access, race and ethnicity is associated with use of PrEP medication among MSM.

The independent variables from above hypothesis are:  Socio-economic status (SES), age, educational attainment, employment status, health care access, race and ethnicity. The dependent variable is the formal/informal use of PrEP. Descriptive statistics was conducted to generate frequency distribution table for the independent variables to show the frequencies and percentages of each demographic group. The values of the independent variable was cross-tabulated with the values of the dependent variable and binary logistic regression will be conducted to determine the association between each independent variable and the dependent variable. The concept of odds ratio (EXP (B), the Sig (p-value) and 95% confidence internal (95% CI) was used to interpret the presence or absent of an association between each independent variable and the dependent variable.

**Hypothesis 3**

*Ho*3: Socio-economic status (SES), age, educational attainment, employment status, health care access, illicit drug use, insertive or receptive anal dominant position, race and ethnicity is not associated with risky sexual behavior among MSM.

*Ha*3: Socio-economic status (SES), age, educational attainment, employment status, health care access, illicit drug use, insertive or receptive anal dominant position, race and ethnicity is associated with risky sexual behavior among MSM.

The independent variables from above hypothesis are: Socio-Economic Status (SES), age, educational attainment, employment status, health care access, illicit drug use, insertive or receptive anal dominant position, and race/ethnicity. The dependent variable is risky sexual behavior. Descriptive statistics was conducted to generate frequency distribution table for the independent variables to show the frequencies and percentages of each independent variable. The values of the independent variable was cross-tabulated with the values of the dependent variable and binary logistic regression was conducted to determine the association between each independent variable and the dependent variable. The concept of odds ratio (EXP (B), the Sig (p-value) and 95% confidence internal (95% CI) was used to interpret the presence or absent of an association between each independent variable and the dependent variable.

**Threats to Validity**

According to Cohall, et al. (2011), younger participants are more likely to be proficient in computer skills and more knowledgeable with web-based survey structure and language and therefore more likely to complete web-based survey compared to older participants and this was true for this study. Also, this study is in agreement with the notion that people of higher socio-economic class are more likely to have access to computers and the internet compared to people of low socio-economic class and therefore more likely to complete online survey questions (Cohall et al., 2011). Therefore, selection and non-response biases occurred in this study, especially when the answers of those who responded to the survey questions were different from potential answers of those who did not respond to the survey questions (Hunter, 2012). This threatened the internal validity of this study. Also, non-response contributed to the low sample size which also threatened the internal validity of this study (Hunter, 2012). These internal validity threats were partially addressed by ensuring that participants had the ability to skip any question if they wish to do so and by allowing participants the opportunity to save their answers and then return at a later time to complete the survey. Also, the cross-sectional design and convenience sampling method selected for this study helped to reduce restrictions to interested participants and allow reasonable time window for more participant to complete the survey questions. Follow up email reminder was sent to participants who did not respond after two weeks to encourage them to complete the survey.

The convenience sampling method selected for this study contributed to selection bias and over representation of certain demographic groups and under representation of other groups (Hunter, 2012). Because of the absence of random sampling methodology, the results of the study was not representative of the study population and therefore the external validity and generalizability of the results was compromised. The external validity issues emanating from convenience sampling methodology was reduced by increasing the sample size through recruitment of more participants above the estimated sample size (Hunter, 2011). Under representation of certain demographic groups was reduced by distributing survey notices and advertisement through social organizations that provide social services to diversified population of potential participants. This created both awareness and more opportunities to underserved groups to participate in the survey.

## Ethical Issues

Demographic and behavioral data of research participants was collected using web-based survey. As such, protecting the privacy and confidentiality of respondents' personal information and obtaining properly executed informed consent posed ethical concerns (University of Massachusetts, 2013). Breach of privacy and anonymity of participants could have occurred during data transmission of the survey questions (Survey Monkey, 2014). Also, it is possible that a hacker may have traced the IP address and websites visited by the respondents prior to accessing the survey website and then tracked the respondent's online activities on the internet for other purposes (Survey Monkey, 2014). Since web-based information technology is constantly evolving, it may be difficult to ensure 100% privacy and confidentiality during all data transmission during web-based surveys (Survey Monkey, 2014). Survey Monkey was contracted to deliver the survey for this study and the organization has inbuilt security checks to ensure anonymity, privacy and confidentiality of respondents. The organization makes use of Secure Sockets Layer (SSL) encryption technology to secure connections between a client and the server and this ensured secured data download and transmission that protected respondents' private information and IP address (Survey Monkey, 2014).

In Online surveys, breach of privacy could also occur when respondents are recruited to complete web-based surveys without prior informed consent of potential participants or inadequately executed informed consent process (University of Massachusetts, 2013). Because of the distance between the participants and the investigator, it was difficult for the respondents in this study to ask questions regarding their concerns and purpose of the study prior to signing the electronic consent form (University of Massachusetts, 2013). Also, it is possible that some respondents did not understand the details of the electronic consent form and did not take time to read the form before signing it (University of Massachusetts, 2013). Even though there is no one standardized web-based consent form, the electronic consent form created for this study ensured adequate execution by making sure that the language verbiage is written in grade 3 English language standard. The consent form was signed by all interested participants before having access to the survey questions. The consent form clearly indicated the inclusion and exclusion criteria to discourage ineligible participants from signing the consent form. Also, processes deployed to ensure anonymity and privacy was provided in the consent form as well as the risks, benefits and limitations of the inbuilt data security tool. Agreeing to sign the consent form allowed access to the survey questions, while disagreeing to sign the consent form ended the survey.

## Summary

Chapter 3 provided detailed description of this quantitative, cross-sectional, web-based primary data analysis of the role of preexposure prophylaxis and socio-demographic factors on sexual risk behavior among MSM residing in the United States. Procedures for data collection, measurement scales for the dependent and independent variables, validity issues of the research method and ethical concerns of the data

collection process were addressed. Also, procedures for the interpretation of research

results and key parameter estimates such as odds ratio, confidence interval and

probability estimates were addressed in Chapter 3. Chapter 4 provide detailed

descriptions of the results and findings of this study, including the descriptive and

inferential statistics, as well as the criteria for the interpretation of significant results were

applicable.

Chapter 4: Results

## Introduction

The purpose of this study was to determine the potential association between sociodemographic factors and the use of preexposure prophylaxis for HIV prevention and sexual risk behavior among MSM in the United States using primary data analysis. The rising rate of new HIV infections among MSM population and the introduction of pre-exposure prophylaxis to augment behavioral intervention programs drew awareness to potential safe sex compromise that might blunt the possible gains of the use of pre-exposure prophylaxis. Findings from this study are expected to augment to the current scarce literature on the possible association between PrEP and sexual risk behavior among MSM under natural conditions devoid of controlled clinical trial environment in previous studies. Also, conflicting findings on the association between Sociodemographic characteristics and sexual risk behavior among MSM was addressed for purposes of preventive targeting of at risk MSM groups. The research questions that guided this research inquiry and the hypotheses created from the research questions were as follows:

RQ1: Is the use of prophylactic antiretroviral medications associated with risky sexual behavior among MSM?

*Ho*1: Prophylactic antiretroviral medication is not associated with risky sexual behavior among MSM.

*Ha*1: Prophylactic antiretroviral medication is associated with risky sexual behavior among MSM.

Significance Level: Reject *Ho*1 if p-value < 0.05

RQ2: Do socio-economic status (SES), age, educational attainment, employment status, health care access, race and ethnicity predict use of PrEP among MSM?

*H*o2: Socio-economic status (SES), age, educational achievement, employment status, health care access, race and ethnicity is not associated with use of PrEP medication among MSM.

*H*a2: Socio-economic status (SES), age, educational attainment, employment status, health care access, race and ethnicity is associated with use of PrEP medication among MSM.

Significance Level: Reject *H*o2 if p-value < 0.05

RQ3: Do socio-economic status (SES), age, educational attainment, employment status, health care access, illicit drug use, insertive or receptive anal dominant position, race and ethnicity predict risky sexual behavior among MSM?

*H*o3: Socio-economic status (SES), age, educational achievement, employment status, health care access, illicit drug use, insertive or receptive anal dominant position, race and ethnicity is not associated with risky sexual behavior among MSM.

*H*a3: Socio-economic status (SES), age, educational achievement, employment status, health care access, illicit drug use, insertive or receptive anal dominant position, race and ethnicity is associated with risky sexual behavior among MSM.

Significance Level: Reject *H*o3 if p-value < 0.05

Chapter 4 provides detailed information on the data collection time frame and response rate to the survey by each of the demographic groups represented in the study sample. The differences between the data collection plans proposed in Chapter 3 and the data collection plans implemented in Chapter 4 are highlighted to expose discrepancies between them. Statistical analytical findings are reported in this chapter and findings discovered during the analysis were organized to provide answers to each research question and hypothesis. Additional statistical analysis that was during analysis of the main hypotheses is also discussed. Tables generated during statistical analysis are presented to simplified understanding of the statistical results at a glance. Finally, summary of the answers to all the research questions and hypotheses as well as the statistical significance of the results are discussed.

## Recruitment and Response Rate

Participants for this study were solicited by emails sent to MSM residing in United States. The e-mails contained custom web-link that was created to re-direct potential participants to the survey page; and by clicking on the link or copying and pasting the link to the web browser, the subjects were able to access and complete the survey. The recruitment period lasted for 2 months. The first week of the deployment of the survey showed an average recruitment of two participants who completed the survey per day, while the second week showed an average recruitment of 10 participants who completed survey questions per day. At the end of eight weeks from the time of initial recruitment, 350 participants who completed the survey questions were Screened. Screening declined to zero at the middle of 8 weeks with zero response rate to the survey questions; and remained zero thereafter until the survey was discontinued for final analysis.

Initially, the target population for this study was MSM residing in New York and California States and subjects recruitment started out from these two states. After 3 weeks of data collection, 74 participants were recruited and subject's response rate to the survey questions declined to zero. Preliminary analysis of the data collected showed that only two participants were actively using PrEP for HIV prevention. This necessitated a review of the target population and study procedure. In order to enhance the chances of recruiting more MSM who were actively taking PrEP medication for HIV prevention, the target population was expanded to include all 50 States in United States of America. Application for procedure change was solicited from the Walden IRB and approval was granted (IRB approval #09-16-14-0349361).

## Data Collation

Participants responses to the survey questions was downloaded from Survey Monkey software in excel, pdf and SPSS files and saved in computer hard drive. The data and information in the three files were verified for quality by comparing the information in the three files for consistency and similarity. Eight participants were eliminated because they failed to indicate their country of residence, thereby resulting in 342 participants who qualified to be included in the final statistical analysis. There were 19 questions in the survey and each question had multiple options representing 19 variables. The options to each question was represented with numerical number such as 0, 1, 3, 4… etc. After manually verifying the data for all the 342 participants, variable names, variable labels and variable values was created in the variable view of the SPSS software. The data for each variable for all the 342 participants was entered into the data view of the SPSS software.

## Descriptive Statistics

The participants recruited for this study were MSM who volunteered to complete web-based survey and who resides in United States of America. Table 1 shows the age distribution of the participants. Participants who were 45-54 years old and who signed web-based informed consent form volunteered most compared to other age groups (105 subjects or 30.6%), followed closely by those who belonged to 55-64 age range (97 subjects or 28.4%). Those who belonged to age range of 22-34, 35-44, 65 and over consisted of 34 subjects (9.9%), 37 subjects (10.8%), and 61 subjects (18.0%) respectively. Six subject (1.7%) were aged 21 and under while 2 subject (0.6%) refused to disclose their age.

Table 1

*Age Distribution of Participants*

| Age | Frequency | (%) |
| --- | --- | --- |
| 21 and under | 6 | 1.7 |
| 22-34 | 34 | 9.9 |
| 35-44 | 37 | 10.8 |
| 45-54 | 105 | 30.6 |
| 55-64 | 97 | 28.4 |
| 65 and over | 61 | 18.0 |
| Refused to answer | 2 | 0.6 |
| Total | 342 | 100.0 |

Table 2 showed that participants with any post-graduate education and some college degree made up to about 66% of the subjects recruited for the study (110 or

32.1% and 116 or 33.1% respectively). Also, 94 participants with bachelor's degree (27.4%) and 18 participants with grade 12 or GED (5.2%) were recruited.

Table 2

*Educational Achievement of Participants*

| Education | Frequency | (%) |
|---|---|---|
| Never Attended School | 0 | 0 |
| Grade 1-8 | 0 | 0 |
| Grade 9-11 | 4 | 1.2 |
| Grade 12 or GED | 18 | 5.2 |
| Some College | 110 | 32.1 |
| Bachelor's Degree | 94 | 27.4 |
| Any Post-Graduate Studies | 116 | 33.9 |
| Total | 342 | 100 |

As displayed in Table 3, majority of the subjects recruited for this study have full-time employment (187 or 54.5.5%), while those who have part-time employment consisted of 27 participants (9.9%). Also, 85 (24.8%) of the subjects were retired. 9 (2.6) participant were full time students and 2 (0.6%) were home makers. 10 (2.9%) participants were unemployed and 17 (5.0%) were unable to work for health reasons.

Table 3

*Employment Status of Participants*

| Employment Category | Frequency | (%) |
|---|---|---|
| Employed Full Time | 187 | 54.5 |
| Employed Part Time | 27 | 7.9 |
| A Home Maker | 2 | 0.6 |
| Full-Time Student | 9 | 2.6 |
| Retired | 85 | 24.8 |
| Unable to work | 17 | 5.0 |
| Unemployed | 10 | 2.9 |
| Other | 2 | 0.6 |
| Refused to answer | 3 | 0.9 |
| Total | 342 | 100 |

The income category of research participants as displayed in Table 4 shows that the majority of volunteers who completed the study survey belonged to high income bracket ($75,000 or more) and they made up to 28.6% of the study population. The income of the remaining 71.4% of the study population was somewhat evenly distributed across all income brackets captured during the survey.

Table 4

*Income Bracket of Participants*

| Income | Frequency | (%) |
|---|---|---|
| $0 - $4,999 | 10 | 2.9 |
| $5,000 - $9,999 | 5 | 1.5 |
| $10,000 - $12,499 | 6 | 1.7 |
| $12,500 - $14,999 | 8 | 2.3 |
| $15,000 - $19,999 | 15 | 4.4 |
| $20,000 - $24,999 | 21 | 6.1 |
| $25,000 - $29,999 | 15 | 4.4 |
| $30,000 - $34,999 | 18 | 5.2 |
| $35,000 - $39,999 | 23 | 6.7 |
| $40,000 - $49,999 | 33 | 9.6 |
| $50,000 - $59,999 | 32 | 9.3 |
| $60,000 - $74,999 | 39 | 11.4 |
| $75,000 or More | 98 | 28.6 |
| Other | 2 | 0.6 |
| Refused to answer | 16 | 4.7 |
| Don't know | 1 | 0.3 |
| Total | 342 | 100 |

In Table 5 below, participants who identified their race as white constitutes the majority of the study subjects (89.5%). The remaining 10.5% of the subjects were somewhat evenly distributed among groups who identified themselves as American Indian, Asian, African-American and Hispanic races.

Table 5

*Race Distribution of Participants*

| Race | Frequency | (%) |
|---|---|---|
| American Indian | 6 | 1.7 |
| Asian | 7 | 2.0 |
| Black or African American | 9 | 2.6 |
| Hispanic | 9 | 2.6 |
| Native Hawaiian | 0 | 0 |
| White | 307 | 89.5 |
| Refused to answer | 4 | 1.2 |
| Total | 342 | 100.0 |

Descriptive statistics displayed in Table 6 show that 72.9 % of the research Subjects identified their HIV status as negative, while 14% of the subject identified their HIV status as HIV positive. 5.8% of the subject declined to disclose their HIV status while 2.9% of the subjects did not know their HIV status. 3.8% of the study subjects never obtained results of their HIV tests.

Table 6

*HIV Status of Research Subjects*

| HIV Test Results | Frequency | (%) |
| --- | --- | --- |
| Negative | 250 | 72.9 |
| Positive | 48 | 14.0 |
| Never obtained result | 13 | 3.8 |
| Indeterminate | 1 | 0.3 |
| Refused to Answer | 20 | 5.8 |
| Don't Know | 10 | 2.9 |
| Total | 342 | 100 |

As shown in Table 7, 53 (15.5%) of the subjects use alcohol during sex while 12 (3.5%) use any form of drugs during sex. Also, 11 (3.2%) of the subjects use both drugs and alcohol during sex. Majority of the subjects (243 (70.8%) did not use drug or alcohol during sex. However, 4.7% and 2% of the subjects declined to answer and don't know if they used drugs or alcohol during sex respectively.

Table 7

*Substance Use during Sex*

| Substance | Frequency | (%) |
|---|---|---|
| Alcohol | 53 | 15.5 |
| Drugs | 12 | 3.5 |
| Both alcohol & drugs | 11 | 3.2 |
| No Drugs or Alcohol | 243 | 70.8 |
| Refused to answer | 16 | 4.7 |
| Don't know | 7 | 2.0 |
| Total | 342 | 100.0 |

In Table 8, 317 (92.7%) of the study participants have health insurance coverage while 22 (6.4%) of the subjects have no health insurance coverage. 2 (0.6%) subjects and 1 (0.3%) subject failed to disclose if they had health insurance coverage.

Table 8

*Health Care Access of Study Subjects*

| Health Insurance Coverage | Frequency | (%) |
|---|---|---|
| No | 22 | 6.4 |
| Yes | 317 | 92.7 |
| Refused to Answer | 1 | 0.3 |
| Don't Know | 2 | 0.6 |
| Total | 342 | 100.0 |

**Statistical Assumptions**

Logistic regression was used to analyze the data collected during this study. The consideration for the choice of logistic regression was due to the nonrandom sampling method (Convenience sampling) used to collect web-based data from research subjects. Logistic regression does not require linear relationship between dependent and independent variables and therefore does not need to meet the assumptions of other statistical analytical methods (Statistical Solutions, 2014). Also, logistic regression can handle many kinds of relationships because it deploys a non-linear log transformation to the expected odds ratio ((Statistical Solutions, 2014).

## Data Analysis and Results

The data collected during this study was analyzed using statistical Package for Social Sciences (SPSS) version 20.1. Descriptive statistical analysis was used to appropriately characterize the independent and dependent variables for each research question; and inferential statistics (binary/multiple logistic regression) was deployed to test for any association between the independent and the dependent variables.

### Research Question 1

The first research question that guided this research inquiry is stated as follows:

Is the use of prophylactic antiretroviral medications associated with risky sexual behavior among MSM?

The hypotheses developed from above research question include:

$Ho1$: Prophylactic antiretroviral medication is not associated with risky sexual behavior among MSM.

*Ha*1: Prophylactic antiretroviral medication is associated with risky sexual

behavior among MSM.

Significance Level: Reject *Ho*1 if p-value < 0.05

The independent variable associated with the first research hypothesis was the use

of antiretroviral medication by MSM after sexual encounter. The independent variable

data was collected using the HIV prophylaxis question in the survey tool completed by

the subjects. The HIV prophylaxis questionnaire states as follows: If your HIV test is

negative, in the past 12 months, have you taken anti-HIV medicines before or after sex

because you thought it would keep you from getting HIV? The independent variable

value for the predictor variable was captured in the variable view of the SPSS software

as: No = 1, Yes = 2, refused to answer = 7, and don't know = 9. Tables 9 and 10

displayed the descriptive statistics of the independent variables.

Table 9

*Use of Preexposure Prophylaxis after Sex*

| Used PrEP | Frequency | (%) |
|---|---|---|
| No | 287 | 83.7 |
| Yes | 5 | 1.5 |
| Refused to Answer | 33 | 9.6 |
| Don't Know | 17 | 5.0 |
| Total | 342 | 100.0 |

Table 10

*Use of Preexposure Prophylaxis before Sex*

| Used PrEP | Frequency | (%) |
|---|---|---|
| No | 279 | 81.7 |
| Yes | 11 | 3.2 |
| Refused to Answer | 33 | 9.6 |
| Don't Know | 19 | 5.5 |
| Total | 342 | 100.0 |

The dependent variable associated with the first research hypothesis was the risky sexual behavior adopted by the subjects. Risky sexual behavior is defined as sexual encounter with multiple partners or lack of use condom during receptive/insertive anal sex or both. The dependent variable data was collected using the risky sexual behavior questions in the survey tool completed by the subjects. The risky sexual behavior questionnaire states as follows: During the past 12 months when you were having a sexual relationship with your partner, did you have sex with other people or use condom during insertive/receptive anal sex? The dependent variable value was captured in the variable view of the SPSS software as: No = 1, Yes = 2, refused to answer = 7, and don't know = 9. Table 11 displays the output logistic regression statistics of the independent and dependent variables.

Table 11

*Logistic Regression of PrEP and Adoption of Multiple Sexual Partner*

| PrEP | B | S.E | Wald | df | Sig | EXP (B) | 95% C.I. Lower | 95% C.I. Upper |
|---|---|---|---|---|---|---|---|---|
| PREP-B | 1.75 | 1.15 | 2.33 | 1 | 0.13 | 5.75 | 0.61 | 54.43 |
| PREP-A | -2.34 | 1.56 | 2.24 | 1 | 0.13 | 0.10 | 0.01 | 2.06 |
| Constant | -0.58 | 0.13 | 20.39 | 1 | 0.00 | 0.56 | | |

*Note. PREP-B = Preexposure prophylaxis before sex. PREP-A = Preexposure prophylaxis after sex*

Subjects who use HIV preexposure prophylaxis before sex were 5.75 times as likely to adopt multiple sexual partner behavior as participants who did not use preexposure prophylaxis before sex. Odds ratio was not statistically significant because 95% confidence interval (0.61, 54.43) included/contained 1.0 and the p-value (0.13) is > 0.05. Also, subjects who use HIV preexposure prophylaxis after sex were 0.10 times as likely to adopt multiple sexual partner behavior as participants who did not use preexposure prophylaxis after sex. Odds ratio was not statistically significant because 95% confidence interval (0.01, 2.06) included/contained 1.0 and the p-value (0.13) is > 0.05. *Ho*1 which states that Prophylactic antiretroviral medication is not associated with risky sexual behavior among MSM was accepted while *Ha*1 which states that Prophylactic antiretroviral medication is associated with risky sexual behavior among MSM was rejected.

Table 12

*Logistic Regression of PrEP and Avoidance of Condom during Insertive Anal Sex*

| PREP | B | S.E | Wald | df | Sig | EXP (B) | 95% C.I Lower | 95% C.I. Upper |
|---|---|---|---|---|---|---|---|---|
| PREP-B | 0.90 | 0.94 | 0.91 | 1 | 0.34 | 2.46 | 0.39 | 15.68 |
| PREP-A | -0.49 | 1.22 | 0.16 | 1 | 0.69 | 0.62 | 0.06 | 6.68 |
| Constant | -0.66 | 0.14 | 22.61 | 1 | 0.00 | 0.52 | | |

Subjects who use HIV preexposure prophylaxis before sex were 2.46 times as likely to adopt insertive anal sex without condom as participants who did not use preexposure prophylaxis before sex. Odds ratio was not statistically significant because 95% confidence interval (0.39, 15.68) included/contained 1.0 and the P-Value (0.34) is > 0.05. Also, subjects who use HIV preexposure prophylaxis after sex were 0.62 times as likely to adopt insertive anal sex without condom as participants who did not use pre-exposure prophylaxis before sex. Odds ratio was not statistically significant because 95% confidence interval (0.06, 6.68) included/contained 1.0 and the p-value (0.69) is > 0.05. *Ho*1 which states that Prophylactic antiretroviral medication is not associated with risky sexual behavior among MSM was accepted while *Ha*1 which states that Prophylactic antiretroviral medication is associated with risky sexual behavior among MSM was rejected.

Table 13

*Logistic Regression of PrEP Use and Avoidance of Condom during Receptive Anal Sex*

| PREP | B | S.E | Wald | df | Sig | EXP (B) | 95% C.I. Lower | 95% C.I. Upper |
|---|---|---|---|---|---|---|---|---|
| PREP-B | 0.29 | 0.85 | 0.12 | 1 | 0.73 | 1.34 | 0.26 | 7.02 |
| PREP-A | -0.23 | 1.14 | 0.04 | 1 | 0.84 | 0.80 | 0.09 | 7.45 |
| Constant | -0.42 | 0.14 | 9.26 | 1 | 0.00 | 0.66 | | |

Subjects who use HIV preexposure prophylaxis before sex were 1.34 times as likely to adopt receptive anal sex without condom as participants who did not use preexposure prophylaxis before sex. Odds ratio was not statistically significant because 95% confidence interval (0.26, 7.02) included/contained 1.0 and the p-value (0.73) is > 0.05. Subjects who use HIV preexposure prophylaxis after sex were 0.80 times as likely to adopt receptive anal sex without condom as participants who did not use pre-exposure prophylaxis after sex. Odds ratio was not statistically significant because 95% confidence interval (0.09, 7.45) included/contained 1.0 and the p-value (0.84) is > 0.05. *Ho*1 which states that Prophylactic antiretroviral medication is not associated with risky sexual behavior among MSM was accepted while *Ha*1 which states that Prophylactic antiretroviral medication is associated with risky sexual behavior among MSM was rejected.

**Research Question 2**

The second research question that guided this research inquiry is stated as follows:

Do socio-economic status (SES), age, educational attainment, employment status, health care access, race and ethnicity predict use of PrEP among MSM?

The hypotheses developed from above research question include:

*Ho*2: Socio-economic status (SES), age, educational attainment, employment status, health care access, race and ethnicity is not associated with use of PrEP medication among MSM.

*Ha*2: Socio-economic status (SES), age, educational attainment, employment status, health care access, race and ethnicity is associated with use of PrEP medication among MSM.

Significance Level: Reject *Ho*2 if p-value < 0.05

The dependent variable associated with the second research hypothesis was the risky sexual behavior adopted by the subjects. Risky sexual behavior for research question 2 is defined as sexual encounter with multiple partners because more subjects adopted multiple sexual partner compared to those who failed to use condom during anal sex. The dependent variable data was collected using the risky sexual behavior questions in the survey tool completed by the subjects. The risky sexual behavior questionnaire states as follows: During the past 12 months when you were having a sexual relationship with your partner, did you have sex with other people? The dependent variable value was captured in the variable view of the SPSS software as: No = 1, Yes = 2.

Table 14 displays the descriptive statistics of educational achievements of study participants who are actively on PrEP medication for HIV prevention, while table 15 shows the output logistic regression statistics of educational achievements predicting the adoption of PrEP. Subjects who had Grade 12/GED, and any post-graduate education had statistically significant odds ratio because 95% confidence interval (0.00, 0.12; and 0.00, 0.27 respectively) did not contain 1.0 and the p-values (0.01, 0.03) is < 0.05. *Ho*2 which states that educational attainment is not associated with the use of PrEP medication among MSM was rejected, while *Ha*2 which states that educational attainment is associated with use of PrEP medication among MSM was accepted.

Table 14

*Educational Achievement of PrEP Users*

| Education | Frequency | (%) |
|---|---|---|
| Grade 12 or GED | 2 | 18.2 |
| Bachelor's Degree | 1 | 9.1 |
| Any Post-graduate | 4 | 36.4 |
| Refused to answer | 4 | 36.4 |
| Total | 11 | 100.0 |

Table 15

*Logistic Regression of Educational Achievement Predicting PrEP Use*

| Education | B | S.E | Wald | df | Sig | EXP (B) | 95% C.I. Lower | 95% C.I. Upper |
|---|---|---|---|---|---|---|---|---|
| Grade 12 | -5.20 | 1.59 | 10.79 | 1 | 0.01 | 0.005 | 0.00 | 0.12 |
| Bachelor's | -3.6 | 1.33 | 7.34 | 1 | 0.07 | 0.03 | 0.002 | 0.32 |
| Post-Grad | -3.90 | 1.33 | 8.70 | 1 | 0.03 | 0.20 | 0.002 | 0.27 |
| Constant | 0.69 | 1.23 | 0.32 | 1 | 0.57 | 2.00 | | |

Table 16 displays the descriptive statistics of age distribution of study participants who were actively on PrEP medication for HIV prevention, while table 17 shows the output logistic regression statistics of age distribution predicting the adoption of PrEP. Odd ratio for all age category was not statistically significant because 95% confidence interval contained 1.0 and the p-values (1.00) is >0.05. *Ho*2 which states that age is not associated with the use of PrEP medication among MSM was accepted, while *Ha*2 which states that age is associated with use of PrEP medication among MSM was rejected.

Table 16

*Age Distribution of PrEP Users*

| Age (Years) | Frequency | (%) |
| --- | --- | --- |
| 22-34 | 1 | 9.1 |
| 35-44 | 4 | 36.4 |
| 45-54 | 3 | 27.3 |
| 55-64 | 3 | 27.3 |
| Total | 11 | 100.0 |

Table 17

*Logistic Regression of Age Predicting PrEP Use*

| Age | B | S.E | Wald | df | Sig | EXP (B) | 95% C.I. Lower | 95% C.I. Upper |
| --- | --- | --- | --- | --- | --- | --- | --- | --- |
| 22-34 | 19.10 | 28421.17 | 0.00 | 1 | 1.00 | 208451022.2 | 0.00 | . |
| 35-44 | 17.91 | 28421.17 | 0.00 | 1 | 1.00 | 59833163.79 | 0.00 | . |
| 45-54 | 17.91 | 28421.17 | 0.00 | 1 | 1.00 | 59833163.79 | 0.00 | . |
| 55-64 | 0.00 | 28973.07 | 0.00 | 1 | 1.00 | 1.00 | 0.00 | . |
| Constant | -21.20 | 28421.17 | 0.00 | 1 | 0.00 | 1.00 | | |

Table 18 shows the descriptive statistics of race distribution of study participants who were actively on PrEP medication for HIV prevention, while table 19 shows the output logistic regression statistics of race distribution predicting the adoption of PrEP. Odds ratio for all race category was not statistically significant because 95% confidence interval contained 1.0 and the P-Values (1.00) is >0.05. $Ho2$ which states that race is not associated with the use of PrEP medication among MSM was accepted, while $Ha2$ which states that race is associated with use of PrEP medication among MSM was rejected.

Table 18

*Race Distribution of PrEP Users*

| Race | Frequency | (%) |
|---|---|---|
| African-American | 4 | 36.4 |
| Hispanic | 1 | 9.1 |
| White | 5 | 45.5 |
| Refused to answer | 1 | 9.1 |
| Total | 11 | 100.0 |

Table 19

*Logistic Regression of Race Predicting PrEP Use*

| Race | B | S.E | Wald | df | Sig | EXP (B) | 95% C.I. Lower | 95% C. I. Upper |
|---|---|---|---|---|---|---|---|---|
| Blacks | 19.26 | 23205.02 | 0.00 | 1 | 1.00 | 230779330.5 | 0.00 | . |
| Hispanic | 17.26 | 23205.02 | 0.00 | 1 | 1.00 | 31307273.52 | 0.00 | . |
| White | 20.51 | 23205.02 | 0.00 | 1 | 1.00 | 807727656.8 | 0.00 | . |
| Constant | -21.20 | 23205.02 | 0.00 | 1 | 1.00 | 0.00 | | |

Table 20 shows the descriptive statistics of income distribution of study participants who were actively on PrEP medication for HIV prevention. Also, table 21 shows the output logistic regression statistics of income distribution predicting the adoption of PrEP. Odds ratio for all income category was not statistically significant because 95% confidence interval contained 1.0 and the p-values (1.00) is >0.05. The *Ho2* which states that income is not associated with the use of PrEP medication among MSM was accepted, while *Ha2* which states that income is associated with use of PrEP medication among MSM was rejected.

Table 20

*Income Category of PrEP Users*

| Income ($) | Frequency | Percent (%) |
| --- | --- | --- |
| 20,000-24,999 | 1 | 9.1 |
| 25,000-29,999 | 1 | 9.1 |
| 30,000-34,999 | 1 | 9.1 |
| 35,000-39,999 | 1 | 9.1 |
| 60,000-74,999 | 1 | 9.1 |
| 75,000 or more | 6 | 54.6 |
| Total | 11 | 100 |

Table 21

*Logistic Regression of Income Predicting PrEP Use*

| Income | B | S.E | Wald | df | Sig | EXP (B) | 95% C.I. Lower | 95% C.I. Upper |
| --- | --- | --- | --- | --- | --- | --- | --- | --- |
| 20,000-24,999 | 18.37 | 40193.55 | 0.00 | 1 | 1.00 | 95028927.66 | 0.00 | . |
| 75,000 or more | 18.41 | 40193.55 | 0.00 | 1 | 1.00 | 98505595.74 | 0.00 | . |
| Constant | -21.20 | 40193.55 | 0.00 | 1 | 1.00 | 0.00 | | |

Table 22 displays the descriptive statistics of employment status of study participants

who were actively on PrEP medication for HIV prevention, while Table 23 shows the

output logistic regression statistics of employment status predicting the adoption of PrEP.

Subjects who work full time and those who are unable to work due to health reasons had statistically significant odds ratio because 95% confidence interval (2.31, 106.74; and 2.31, 59.96 respectively) did not contain 1.0 and the p-values (0.005, 0.002) is < 0.05. *H*o2 which states that employment status is not associated with the use of PrEP medication among MSM was rejected, while *H*a2 which states that employment status is associated with use of PrEP medication among MSM was accepted.

Table 22

*Employment Status of PrEP Users*

| Employment | Frequency | (%) |
| --- | --- | --- |
| Employed full time | 4 | 36.4 |
| Employed part-time | 1 | 9.1 |
| Full time student | 2 | 18.2 |
| Unable to work | 3 | 27.3 |
| Unemployed | 1 | 9.1 |
| Total | 11 | 100 |

Table 23

*Logistic Regression of Employment Predicting PrEP Use*

| Employ | B | S.E | Wald | df | Sig | EXP (B) | 95% C.I. Lower | 95% C.I. Upper |
| --- | --- | --- | --- | --- | --- | --- | --- | --- |
| Full Time | 2.75 | 0.98 | 2.93 | 1 | 0.005 | 15.70 | 2.31 | 106.74 |
| Unable to work | 2.47 | 0.83 | 8.82 | 1 | 0.003 | 11.76 | 2.31 | 59.96 |
| Constant | -3.67 | 0.51 | 52.54 | 1 | 0.00 | 0.25 | | |

Table 24 shows the descriptive statistics of health insurance coverage of study participants who were actively on PrEP medication for HIV prevention. Also, table 25 shows the output logistic regression statistics of health insurance coverage predicting the adoption of PrEP. Odds ratio for health insurance coverage was not statistically significant because 95% confidence interval contained 1.0 and the p-values (0.65) is >0.05. *Ho*2 which states that health insurance is not associated with the use of PrEP medication among MSM was accepted, while *Ha*2 which states that health insurance is associated with use of PrEP medication among MSM was rejected.

Table 24

*Health Care Access of PrEP Users*

| Health Insurance | Frequency | (%) |
|---|---|---|
| Has Insurance | 1 | 9.1 |
| Has no insurance | 10 | 90.9 |
| Total | 11 | 100 |

Table 25

*Logistic Regression of Health Care Access Predicting PrEP Use*

| INSUR | B | S.E | Wald | df | Sig | EXP (B) | 95% C.I. Lower | 95% C.I. Upper |
|---|---|---|---|---|---|---|---|---|
| Insurance | -0.50 | 1.10 | 0.21 | 1 | 0.65 | 0.61 | 0.07 | 5.05 |
| Constant | -2.77 | 1.03 | 7.24 | 1 | 0.07 | 0.063 | | |

**Research Question 3**

The third research question that guided this research inquiry is stated as follows:

Do socio-economic status (SES), age, educational attainment, employment status, health care access, illicit drug use, insertive or receptive anal dominant position, race and ethnicity predict risky sexual behavior among MSM?

The hypotheses developed from above research question include:

*H*o3: Socio-economic status (SES), age, educational attainment, employment status, health care access, illicit drug use, insertive or receptive anal dominant position, race and ethnicity is not associated with risky sexual behavior among MSM.

*H*a3: Socio-economic status (SES), age, educational attainment, employment status, health care access, illicit drug use, insertive or receptive anal dominant position, race and ethnicity is associated with risky sexual behavior among MSM.

Significance Level: Reject *H*o3 if p-value $< 0.05$

The dependent variable associated with the second research hypothesis was the risky sexual behavior adopted by the subjects. Risky sexual behavior is defined as sexual encounter with multiple partners. The dependent variable data was collected using the risky sexual behavior questions in the survey tool completed by the subjects. The risky sexual behavior questionnaire states as follows: During the past 12 months when you were having a sexual relationship with your partner, did you have sex with other people? The dependent variable value was captured in the variable view of the SPSS software as: N0 = 1, Yes = 2, refused to answer = 7, and don't know = 9.

Table 26 shows the output logistic regression statistics of anal sex dominant position and health insurance predicting risky sexual behavior among MSM. Subjects who adopted receptive and insertive anal sex position were about 2 times each as likely to adopt risky sexual behavior. Also, they had statistically significant odds ratio because 95% confidence interval (1.35, 3.61; and 1.28, 3.41 respectively) did not contain 1.0 and the p-values (0.002, 0.003) is < 0.05. *Ho*3 which states that anal sex dominant position is not associated with risky sexual behavior among MSM was rejected, while *Ha*3 which states that anal sex position is associated with risky sexual behavior among MSM was accepted. However, health insurance coverage was not statistically significant because 95% confidence interval (0.77, 7.87) contained 1.0 and the p-values (0.13) is >0.05.

Table 26

*Multiple Logistic Regression of Health Care Access and Anal Sex Position Predicting Sexual Risk Behavior*

| | B | S.E | Wald | df | Sig | EXP (B) | 95% C.I. Lower | 95% C.I. Upper |
|---|---|---|---|---|---|---|---|---|
| Health Insurance | 0.90 | 0.59 | 2.33 | 1 | 0.13 | 2.47 | 0.77 | 7.87 |
| Receptive Anal Sex | 0.79 | 0.25 | 9.94 | 1 | 0.002 | 2.21 | 1.35 | 3.61 |
| Insertive Anal Sex | 0.74 | 0.25 | 8.69 | 1 | 0.003 | 2.09 | 1.28 | 3.41 |
| Constant | -2.18 | 0.62 | 12.53 | 1 | 0.00 | 0.11 | | |

Table 27 shows the output logistic regression statistics of age distribution predicting sexual risk behavior among MSM. Odds ratio for all age category was not statistically significant because 95% confidence interval for all age category contained 1.0 and the p-values for all age category is >0.05. *Ho*3 which states that age is not associated with risky sexual behavior among MSM was accepted, while *Ha3* which states that age is associated with risky sexual behavior among MSM was rejected.

Table 27

*Logistic Regression of Age Predicting Sexual Risk Behavior*

| Age | B | S.E | Wald | df | Sig | EXP (B) | 95% C.I. Lower | 95% C.I. Upper |
|---|---|---|---|---|---|---|---|---|
| ≤ 21 | 1.30 | 1.20 | 1.14 | 1 | 0.29 | 3.64 | 0.34 | 39.01 |
| 22-34 | 0.57 | 1.21 | 0.23 | 1 | 0.64 | 1.77 | 0.17 | 18.86 |
| 35-44 | 0.59 | 1.17 | 0.26 | 1 | 0.61 | 1.81 | 0.18 | 18.09 |
| 45-54 | 0.32 | 1.18 | 0.08 | 1 | 0.78 | 1.38 | 0.14 | 13.85 |
| 55-64 | 0.12 | 1.19 | 0.01 | 1 | 0.92 | 1.13 | 0.11 | 11.68 |
| ≥ 65 | 1.01 | 1.83 | 0.36 | 1 | 0.55 | 3.00 | 0.08 | 107.45 |
| Constant | -1.10 | 1.16 | 0.91 | 1 | 0.34 | 0.33 | | |

Table 28 shows the output logistic regression statistics of race distribution predicting sexual risk behavior among MSM. Odds ratio for all race category was not statistically significant because 95% confidence interval for all race category contained 1.0 and the p-values for all age category is >0.05. *Ho3* which states that race is not associated with risky sexual behavior among MSM was accepted, while *Ha3* which states that race is associated with risky sexual behavior among MSM was rejected.

Table 28

*Logistic Regression of Race Predicting Sexual Risk Behavior*

| Race | B | S.E | Wald | df | Sig | EXP (B) | 95% C.I. Lower | 95% C.I. Upper |
|---|---|---|---|---|---|---|---|---|
| Indian | -0.29 | 1.26 | 0.05 | 1 | 0.82 | 0.75 | 0.64 | 8.83 |
| Asian | -0.29 | 1.26 | 0.05 | 1 | 0.82 | 0.75 | 0.64 | 8.83 |
| Black | 0.63 | 1.13 | 0.31 | 1 | 0.58 | 1.88 | 0.20 | 17.27 |
| Hispanic | -0.23 | 0.92 | 0.06 | 1 | 0.81 | 0.80 | 0.13 | 4.86 |
| White | 0.41 | 1.35 | 0.09 | 1 | 0.77 | 1.50 | 0.11 | 21.31 |
| Constant | -0.41 | 0.91 | 0.20 | 1 | 0.66 | 0.67 | | |

Table 29 shows the output logistic regression statistics of educational achievement distribution predicting sexual risk behavior among MSM. Odds ratio for all education category was not statistically significant because 95% confidence interval for all race category contained 1.0 and the p-values for all age category (1.0) is >0.05. *Ho*3 which states that education is not associated with risky sexual behavior among MSM was accepted, while Ha3 which states that education is associated with risky sexual behavior among MSM was rejected.

Table 29

*Logistic Regression of Educational Achievement Predicting Sexual Risk Behavior*

| EDUC | B | S.E | Wald | df | Sig | EXP (B) | 95% C.I. Lower | 95% C.I. Upper |
|---|---|---|---|---|---|---|---|---|
| 12/GED | 20.41 | 28421.48 | 0.00 | 1 | 1.00 | 734320047.1 | 0.00 | . |
| College | 20.28 | 28421.48 | 0.00 | 1 | 1.00 | 641775602.8 | 0.00 | . |
| Bachelors | 20.61 | 28421.48 | 0.00 | 1 | 1.00 | 894296914.6 | 0.00 | . |
| Any Grad | 20.95 | 28421.48 | 0.00 | 1 | 1.00 | 1259545572.0 | 0.00 | . |
| Constant | -21.20 | 28421.48 | 0.00 | 1 | 1.00 | 0.00 | | |

Table 30 shows the output logistic regression statistics of employment status predicting sexual risk behavior among MSM. Odds ratio for all employment category was not statistically significant because 95% confidence interval for all employment category contained 1.0 and the p-values for all employment category is >0.05. *H*o3 which states that employment status is not associated with risky sexual behavior among MSM was accepted, while *H*a3 which states that employment status is associated with risky sexual behavior among MSM was rejected.

Table 30

*Logistic Regression of Employment Status Predicting Sexual Risk Behavior*

| EMPLOY | B | S.E | Wald | df | Sig | EXP (B) | 95% C.I. Lower | 95% C.I. Upper |
|---|---|---|---|---|---|---|---|---|
| Full-Time | -0.49 | 0.47 | 1.08 | 1 | 0.30 | 0.61 | 0.24 | 1.54 |
| Part-Time | -20.75 | 28420.72 | 0.00 | 1 | 1.00 | 0.00 | 0.00 | . |
| Home-Maker | -0.24 | 0.88 | 0.07 | 1 | 0.79 | 0.79 | 0.14 | 4.41 |
| Student | -0.28 | 0.29 | 0.94 | 1 | 0.33 | 0.76 | 0.43 | 1.33 |
| Retired | -0.46 | 0.61 | 0.57 | 1 | 0.45 | 0.63 | 0.19 | 2.09 |
| Unable to work | 0.05 | 0.66 | 0.01 | 1 | 0.94 | 1.05 | 0.29 | 3.85 |
| Unemployed | 0.45 | 1.42 | 0.10 | 1 | 0.75 | 1.57 | 0.10 | 25.58 |
| Constant | -0.45 | 0.16 | 8.54 | 1 | 0.00 | 0.64 | | |

Table 31 shows the output logistic regression statistics of income bracket predicting sexual risk behavior among MSM. Odds ratio for all income category was not statistically significant because 95% confidence interval for all income category contained 1.0 and the p-values for all income category is >0.05. *Ho*3 which states that income bracket is not associated with risky sexual behavior among MSM was accepted, while *Ha*3 which states that income bracket is associated with risky sexual behavior among MSM was rejected.

Table 31

*Logistic Regression of Income Bracket Predicting Sexual Risk Behavior*

| INCOME ($) | B | S.E | Wald | df | Sig | EXP (B) | 95% C.I. Lower | 95% C.I. Upper |
|---|---|---|---|---|---|---|---|---|
| 0-4,999 | -1.10 | 1.63 | 0.45 | 1 | 0.50 | 0.33 | 0.01 | 8.18 |
| 5,000-9,999 | -0.41 | 1.68 | 0.06 | 1 | 0.81 | 0.67 | 0.03 | 18.06 |
| 10,000-12,499 | 0.41 | 1.68 | 0.06 | 1 | 0.81 | 1.50 | 0.06 | 40.63 |
| 12,500-14,999 | -0.51 | 1.60 | 0.10 | 1 | 0.75 | 0.60 | 0.03 | 13.58 |
| 15,000-19,999 | -0.69 | 1.54 | 0.20 | 1 | 0.65 | 0.50 | 0.02 | 10.25 |
| 20,000-24,999 | -0.85 | 1.50 | 0.32 | 1 | 0.57 | 0.43 | 0.02 | 8.04 |
| 25,000-29,999 | -0.47 | 1.53 | 0.10 | 1 | 0.76 | 0.63 | 0.03 | 12.41 |
| 30,000-34,999 | -2.02 | 1.60 | 1.58 | 1 | 0.21 | 0.13 | 0.01 | 3.08 |
| 35,000-39,999 | -0.92 | 1.49 | 0.38 | 1 | 0.54 | 0.40 | 0.02 | 7.48 |
| 40,000-49,999 | -0.64 | 1.47 | 0.19 | 1 | 0.66 | 0.53 | 0.03 | 9.34 |
| 50,000-59,999 | -0.69 | 1.47 | 0.22 | 1 | 0.64 | 0.50 | 0.03 | 9.34 |
| 60,000-74,999 | -0.45 | 1.46 | 0.10 | 1 | 0.76 | 0.64 | 0.04 | 11.02 |
| $\geq 75,000$ | -0.44 | 1.43 | 0.10 | 1 | 0.76 | 0.64 | 0.04 | 10.61 |
| Constant | 0.00 | 1.41 | 0.00 | 1 | 1.00 | 1.00 | | |

Table 32 shows the output logistic regression statistics of alcohol/drugs predicting sexual risk behavior among MSM.  Odds ratio for alcohol, drugs and alcohol combined with drugs was not statistically significant because 95% confidence alcohol, drugs and alcohol combined with drugs contained 1.0 and the p-values is >0.05. *Ho3* which states that alcohol/drug is not associated with risky sexual behavior among MSM was accepted, while *Ha3* which states that alcohol/drug is associated with risky sexual behavior among MSM was rejected.

Table 32

*Logistic Regression of Alcohol/Drugs Predicting Sexual Risk Behavior*

| Alcohol and Drugs | B | S.E | Wald | df | Sig | EXP (B) | 95% C.I. Lower | 95% C. I. Upper |
|---|---|---|---|---|---|---|---|---|
| Alcohol | 1.19 | 0.70 | 2.94 | 1 | 0.09 | 3.29 | 0.84 | 12.86 |
| Drugs | 0.41 | 0.74 | 0.31 | 1 | 0.58 | 1.51 | 0.36 | 6.36 |
| Alcohol & Drugs | 0.003 | 0.33 | 0.00 | 1 | 0.99 | 1.00 | 0.53 | 1.92 |
| Constant | -0.63 | 0.30 | 4.44 | 1 | 0.04 | 0.53 | | |

### Summary

The potential association between sociodemographic characteristics and preexposure prophylaxis and risky sexual behavior among MSM in United States was assessed in this study. Deploying web-based survey, 342 MSM volunteers were recruited across 50 states in United States. Data collected were analyzed using binary and multiple logistic regressions and the results of the analysis were used to answer the research questions and the three hypotheses developed from the research questions. For RQ1, there were no statistically significant association between HIV preexposure prophylaxis and adoption of sexual risk behavior among MSM who were HIV negative and who use PrEP for HIV prevention. For RQ2, there were statistically significant association between education (any post-graduate education and Grade 12/GED) and the adoption of PrEP for HIV prevention. Also, there were statistically significant association between employment status (full time workers and unable to work due to health reasons) and the adoption of PrEP for HIV prevention. Other demographic factors tested in research question 2 showed no statistically significant association with the adoption of PrEP for HIV prevention. The third research hypothesis that sought to determine the association between sociodemographic characteristics and risky sexual behavior was statistically significant for anal sex dominant (receptive and insertive anal position) and risky sexual behavior. Other sociodemographic factors tested did not show any statistically significant association between the factors and sexual risk behavior. Chapter 5 will provide detailed discussion of the result findings, study limitations, and recommendation for future research. In addition, social change implications based on information and knowledge gained from this study was discussed in chapter 5.

Chapter 5: Discussion, Conclusions, and Recommendations

## Introduction

The purpose of this quantitative, cross-sectional, primary data analysis was to determine the potential association between sociodemographic factors and the use of preexposure prophylaxis for HIV prevention and sexual risk behavior among MSM in United States. The high rate of new HIV infection especially among young MSM and those belonging to minority racial groups needed a new preventive strategy to augment the existing sex education programs. The introduction of preexposure prophylaxis to augment behavioral intervention programs drew attention to improved HIV preventive efficacy, but at the same time raised concerns about the possible increased sexual risk behavior might reduce the gains from using pre-exposure prophylaxis. Findings from this study will help to augment current scarce literature on the association between PrEP and sexual risk behavior. The findings could also be helpful in preventive targeting of at risk MSM population.

The data analyzed during this research study was collected using web-based questionnaire created from sections of the National HIV Behavioral Surveillance System (NHBSS) Questionnaire for MSM and developed by the CDC in collaboration with some local health departments across United States. Data were collected from 342 participants who were recruited online and who completed a 19 question survey; thus, the estimated minimum sample size of 73 was exceeded by 269 subject. Binary and multiple logistic regression were used to test three research hypotheses developed from the research questions.

Results of the statistical test of the first research hypotheses indicated no statistically significant association between HIV preexposure prophylaxis and the adoption of sexual risk behavior among MSM who were HIV negative and who use PrEP for HIV prevention. For the second research hypothesis, there was statistically significant association between education (any post-graduate education and Grade 12/GED) and the adoption of PrEP for HIV prevention. Also, there was a statistically significant association between employment status (full time workers and unable to work due to health reasons) and the adoption of PrEP for HIV prevention. Other demographic factors tested in research hypothesis 2 showed no statistically significant association with the use of PrEP for HIV prevention.   The third research hypothesis which sought to determine the association between sociodemographic characteristics and risky sexual behavior was statistically significant for anal sex dominant (receptive and insertive) position and risky sexual behavior. Other sociodemographic factors tested did not show any statistically significant association between the factors and sexual risk behavior.

## Interpretation of Research Findings

During the course of this research study, the possible association between HIV preexposure prophylaxis and sexual risk behavior among MSM as well as the association between demographic factors and the adoption of preexposure prophylaxis was examined. Also, the potential associations between sociodemographic characteristics and sexual risk behavior among MSM was addressed. The interpretation of the findings from testing the research hypotheses and how the findings converge or diverge from previous studies is described below.

**PrEP and Sexual Risk Behavior**

The relationship between preexposure prophylaxis (PrEP) and sexual risk behavior was tested using binary logistic regression; and the findings showed that the use of HIV medication as preexposure prophylaxis by MSM was not significantly associated with sexual risk behavior. Therefore, *Ho*1 which states that Prophylactic antiretroviral medication is not associated with risky sexual behavior among MSM was accepted while *Ha*1 which states that Prophylactic antiretroviral medication is associated with risky sexual behavior among MSM was rejected. This finding is in alignment with the large multi-center iPrEP clinical trial conducted in many countries that found compelling evidence of efficacy, cost effectiveness and lack of resistance and sexual risk behavior change with the use of PrEP for HIV prevention among study participants (CDC, 2013a; Juusola, Brandeau, Owens & Bendavid, 2012). Also, the finding was similar to the finding by Marcus et al (2013), that there was no evidence of increased sexual risk behavior during the IPrEP study period and immediately post study. On the other hand, the findings from this study is at variance from mixed method study conducted by Brooks et al. (2011). Brooks et al. (2011) found that PrEP use might be associated with increased sexual risk behavior that may predispose to HIV infection. However, the participants (who were not on PrEP medication) indicated likelihood to engage in anal sex without condom or use condom erratically and engage in sexual encounter with individuals who are HIV positive. The methodology and design of Brook's study was based on future projections of intended adoption of PrEP for the prevention of HIV infection that may not exactly translate to the behavior of individuals who are on PrEP medication, as against the methodology used for this study. It is however important to note that this study alone is not sufficient to confirm that PrEP is not associated with risky sexual behavior, but adds to the existing scanty literature in support of the lack of risky sexual behavior among PrEP users.

## PrEP and Sociodemographic Factors

The role of sociodemographic factors in the adoption PrEP for HIV prevention by MSM was tested with binary and multiple logistic regression and the findings showed that employment status (full-time employment and those who were unable to work for health reasons) was associated with the adoption of PrEP for HIV prevention. However, health insurance status, income level and race/ethnicity did not significantly predict the adoption of Preexposure prophylaxis by MSM for the prevention of HIV infection. This findings runs contrary to previous computer simulation studies that suggested that easy health care access may facilitate the adoption of PrEP for HIV prevention (Globus et al, 2013). According to Globus et al. (2013), PrEP acceptability and motivation for adherence may involve free access to PrEP and other support services. Also, the finding of lack of association between race/ethnicity and health insurance access and the adoption of PrEP contradicts the finding by Bauemeister et al. (2014) that postulated that young African American and Latino MSM are less likely to use PrEP if there is lack of free access to PrEP or if they lack health insurance to pay for it. In this study, the reasons for the statistically significant adoption of PrEP by MSM who have full time employment and those who are unable to work for health reasons is unknown especially when health insurance coverage failed to significantly predict the adoption of PrEP for HIV prevention. The erratic findings from this study that showed that low level of educational achievement (Grade 12/GED) and high level of educational achievements (any post-graduate studies) was associated with the adoption of PrEP suggests that the decision to adopt the use of PrEP for HIV prevention may be more complex than social factors alone or in combination.

**Sociodemographic Characteristics and Sexual Risk Behavior**

The relationship between sociodemographic characteristic and sexual risk behavior was tested using binary and multiple logistic regression; and the findings showed that sociodemographic factors such as age, health insurance status, level of education, income level, employment status, and alcohol/drug did not significantly predict risky sexual behavior among MSM contrary to findings from previous studies. According to Hampton et al. (2013), young persons who are less than 30 years are less likely to be exposed to public health preventive program and other sex education programs designed to prevent sexually transmitted diseases including HIV infection. The conflicting finding between this study and previous studies underscores the need to determine if there are other factors in play other than the contribution of age alone to risky sexual behavior. Also, Hampton et al. (2013) and Courtenary-Quirk et al. (2008) alluded to a division among investigators in the link between higher education achievements and risky sexual behavior. The non-significant association between educational achievements and sexual risk behavior discovered from this study will add to the body of existing literature and may help to ignite more research inquiries in order to expand existing knowledge and resolve the divisions among investigators. Also, finding from this study that employment status and income level were not associated with risky sexual behavior is in agreement with previous studies (Rueda et al., 2012). According to Rueda et al. (2012), it is unknown if income level, employment or stable employment status is associated with healthy behavior beyond the quality of life benefits provided by stable income and employment. It was suggested in previous studies that lack of health care access is associated with risky sexual behavior among MSM (McKirnan, Du Bois, Alvy & Jones, 2013). The missed opportunity of HIV prevention awareness, safe sex education and HIV testing that could have occurred when accessing the health care system may contribute to higher risky sexual behavior among MSM (Dorell et al., 2011). Finding from this study contradicts the contribution of the lack of health insurance to the risky sexual behavior of MSM and the reasons for this finding is unknown. Also, previous studies show that cocaine and methamphetamine were the drugs mostly consumed by MSM and these drugs have been hypothesized to be associated with risky sexual behavior and increased HIV infection in the community (Vosburgh, Mansergh, Sullivan, & Purcell, 2012; Dirks et al., 2012). The finding that alcohol and substance use was not significantly associated with sexual risk behavior underscores the need to determine if consumption rate and individual capacity to accommodate drugs played a role in sexual behavior differences among those who use drugs and alcohol. However, finding from this study showed equal statistically significant association between insertive and receptive anal sex dominant position and sexual risk behavior even though previous finding found that those who preferred receptive (bottom) anal dominant positioning were two times more likely to be infected with HIV compared to those who preferred insertive (top) dominant position (Wei & Raymond (2011). These findings show that more studies is needed to determine factors that might also be contributing to high HIV infection rate among bottom dominant position other than sexual behavior differences among the two groups.

**Interpretation of Study findings and HBM**

As previously stated in Chapter 2, the Health Belief Model (HBM) was the theoretical framework selected for this study. The model consists of five elements which include: the perceptions of susceptibility, seriousness, benefit, barriers and self-efficacy (Janz & Becker, 1984). The model had been adapted to provide insights in the relationship between various behaviors and disease transmission especially on the relationship between risky sexual behavior and the transmission of HIV infection (Glanz, Rimer & Lewis, 2002). The perception of susceptibility component is when individuals perceive themselves to be susceptible to the risk of developing diseases and may be motivated to take preventive action based on the negative and severe consequences of the perceived risk (Janz & Becker, 1984). As discussed in Chapter 4, the use of preexposure prophylaxis was not significantly associated with risky sexual behavior among MSM which conform to the construct of the perception of susceptibility. However, it is unknown if other factors contributed to this outcome. Also, the modifiable variables component of the health belief model states that personal perception in the health belief model could be modified by many variables and cues to actions such as education level, skills, past experiences among others (Janz & Becker, 1984). According to Hounton, Carabin & Henderson (2005), structural barriers such as poverty, lack of education, gender inequality and other socio-cultural barriers was used to explain condom efficacy in a population of women at risk of HIV infection when knowledge of mode of infection transmission as well as perception of severity and vulnerability of infections failed to explain behavior change. The findings from this study showed that sociodemographic characteristics such as income, education, employment status among others were not associated with risky sexual behavior. These findings contradicted the notion that sociodemographic characteristics could be used to explain behavior change when other components of the HBM failed to do so.

## Limitations of the Study

A number of limitations were encountered during the execution of this study that posed generalizability issues. There were no Native Hawaiian MSM who volunteered to participate in the study and this skewed the racial composition of study participants in favor of other racial groups (Wright, 2006; Konstan et al., 2005; Andrew, Nonnecke & Preece, 2003). Therefore, the study sample did not reflect the racial composition of United States population and the results of this study may not be generalized to the entire study population. The web-based nature of the participant recruitment prevented the random selection of study subjects; and as such, skewed the selection of research volunteers to mostly those who were middle-aged, upscale and upper-middle class with computer access and computer literacy. These attributes further limited the generalizability and validity of the results (Wright, 2006; Konstan et al., 2005; Andrew, Nonnecke & Preece, 2003). Only 3.2% of the study population was on preexposure prophylaxis for the prevention of HIV. Even though this figure reflects the national figure of PrEP prescriptions for purposes of HIV prevention among MSM (1,274 prescriptions in 2012), the figure was not sufficient to draw explicit conclusion on the association between PrEP and sexual risk behavior (Cairns, 2013). Even though the minimum estimated sample size for this study was 73 participants (actual sample size = 342), higher sample size was anticipated in order to increase the number of MSM on PrEP (Frankfort-Nachmias, & Nachmias, 2008). Higher sample size was however not achieved, thereby adding extra layer of limitations to the generalizability of the results.

## Recommendations

Based on the findings, information, and insights gained during the conduct of this study, it is prudent to make some recommendations for future research. Health care providers who prescribe PrEP for HIV prevention should ensure that patients/clients complete standardized sexual risk behavior questionnaire during every prescription refill visits to the doctor's office (CDC, 2011).   At the end of every year or biannually, the questionnaire should be assessed prospectively in a prospective cohort study that will be ongoing to determine the association of PrEP and risky sexual behavior. In this way, the current lack of sufficient data to accurately determine the relationship between PrEP and sexual behavior changes may be resolved. The difficulty in reaching more minority MSM, especially African American, Hispanic and Hawaiian natives underscores the urgency to recruit minority MSM individuals who have earned the trust of their communities as public health/medical field officers (Association of American Medical Colleges, 2014). In this way, minority MSM could be reached for medical information, education, research and other socio-economic issues that might be contributing negatively to the welfare of the group. A cross-sectional study should be conducted annually to monitor retail pharmacy databases across the country for PrEP prescription in order to determine demographic distribution for PrEP users (Cairns, 2013) This will also help to target at risk MSM who are underserved with PrEP and also to direct PrEP research to demographic groups and areas with available and adequate data.

## Implications for Social Change

Some of the discrimination and homophobia directed towards men who have sex with (MSM) by the public is based on the high risk of HIV infection among MSM communities (Galarneau, 2010; Sowell, 2005). As a result, the desire by much MSM to participate in community social activities such as blood donation, assume role models to youths, engage freely in sports and religious activities is either rejected or greatly diminished (Galarneau, 2010; Sowell, 2005). The result of this research might help to inform programs and policies that could lead to the reduction of HIV risk and infections among MSM; and subsequently help to usher in a positive social change whereby MSM are accepted, respected and free to participate in all social, sporting, humanitarian, and religious activities in their communities.

Also, finding from this study show that minority MSM were relatively under-represented in web-based survey and therefore researchers and public health targeting of this group must involve other methods. Such methods must be well researched to ensure improvement in the participation of minority MSM in public health and research activities (Diaz, 2012). It is advised to recruit, train, and deploy minority MSM as public health field officers who are trusted members of their communities to assist in providing public health services to the underserved minority MSM communities (AAMC, 2014). The penetration of public health activities into minority MSM communities might help to unlock this community from the larger society and bring about integrated social and public health interaction between this community and the larger society (Andrinopoulos & Hembling, 2014).

## Conclusions

The objective of this web-based, quantitative, cross-sectional study was to determine the association between antiretroviral preexposure prophylaxis (PrEP) and sexual risk behavior among MSM who are currently using PrEP for the prevention of

HIV infection in United States of America. Also, this study quantitatively examined the relationship between sociodemographic characteristics and sexual risk behavior among MSM and how PrEP use varies across various groups of MSM. Findings from the study showed that the use of HIV Preexposure prophylaxis was not associated with sexual risk behavior among those MSM who currently use HIV medicines before or after sex to prevent HIV infection. There was however an association between educational achievement and employment status and the adoption of PrEP for HIV prevention among MSM.  The finding of lack of association between PrEP and sexual risk behavior is in agreement with the findings in previous studies. Also, there was no statistically significant association between sociodemographic factors and sexual risk behavior. This finding contradicts previous finding that associated sexual risk behavior with poverty, low education, employment status and age of MSM persons. These findings suggest that the contributing factors to sexual risk behavior among MSM may be more complex than social factors and the use of PrEP. As such, studies related to sexual risk behavior and HIV transmission among MSM should be a continuum until HIV infection in MSM communities is completely prevented.

References

Allen, K. A., Pocock, A. M., Kogan, S. M., Grang, C., Cho, J., Brody, G. H. (n.d.). The influence of perceived discrimination on the risky sexual behavior of rural African American adolescent men. Retrieved from http://www.ncfr.org/sites/default/files/downloads/news/107_ncfr_perceived_discr imination_presentation.pdf

Andrews, D., Nonnecke, B., & Preece, J. (2003). Electronic survey methodology: A case study in reaching hard-to-involve Internet users. *International Journal of Human-Computer Interaction, 16* (2), 185–210. doi:10.1207/S15327590IJHC1602_04

Andrinopoulos, K. & Hembling, J. (2014). Fact sheet: Unlocking health services for MSM and transgender women in San Salvador. Retrieved from http://www.cpc.unc.edu/measure/publications/fs-14-108

Asare, M., Sharma, M., Bernard, A. L., Rojas-Guyler, L., & Wang, L. L. (2013). Using the health belief model to determine safer sexual behavior among African immigrants. *Journal of Health Care for the Poor and Underserved, 24*(1), 120-134

Association of American Medical Colleges. (2014). Minorities in medicine. Retrieved from https://www.aamc.org/students/minorities/

Balaji, A., Bowles, K., Le, B., Paz-Bailey, G., & Oster, A. (2013). High HIV incidence and prevalence and associated factors among young MSM, 2008. *AIDS (London, England), 27*(2), 269-278. doi:10.1097/QAD.0b013e32835ad489

Bangsberg, D. R., Moss, A. R., & Deeks, S. G. (2004). Paradox of adherence and drug

    resistance to HIV antimicrobial therapy. *Journal of Antimicrobial Chemotherapy,*

    *53,* 696-699. doi:10.1093/jac/dkh162

Bauermeister, J., Meanley, S., Pingel, E., Soler, J., & Harper, G. (2013). PrEP awareness

    and perceived barriers among single young men who have sex with men. *Current*

    *HIV Research, 11* (7), 520-527(8)

Bergeson, S., Gray, J., Ehrmantraut, L., Laibson, T., & Hays, R. (2013). Comparing web-

    based with mail survergey administration of the consumer assessment of

    healthcare providers and systems. *Primary Health Care: Open Access, 3,*

    1000032. **doi:10.4172/2167-1079.1000132**

Bize, R., Volkmar, E., Berrut, S., Medico, D., Balthasar, H., Bodenmann, P., Makadon,

    H. (2011). Access to quality primary care for LGBT people. *Revue Medcale*

    *Suisse*, 7(307), 1712-1717.

Bowden, V. R. (2010). Demystifying the research process: cross-sectional

    design. *Pediatric Nursing, 37*(3), 127-128.

Brooks, R. A., Landovitz, R. J., Kaplan, R. L., Lieber, E., Lee, S., & Barkley, T. W.

    (2012). sexual risk behaviors and acceptability of HIV Preexposure prophylaxis

    among HIV-negative gay and bisexual men in serodiscordant relationships: A

    mixed methods study. *AIDS Patient Care & Stds, 26*(2), 87-94.

    doi:10.1089/apc.2011.0283

Cairns, G. (2013). ICAAC 2013: Many Truvada PrEP users are women and young

    people. Retrieved from http://www.hivandhepatitis.com/hiv-prevention/hiv-prep/4289-icaac-2013-many-truvada-prep-users-are-women-and-young-people-survey-finds

Calabrese, S., Earnshaw, V., Underhill, K., Hansen, N., & Dovidio, J. (2014). The impact of patient race on clinical decisions related to prescribing HIV preexposure prophylaxis (PrEP): Assumptions about sexual risk compensation and pmplications for access. *AIDS and Behavior, 18*(2), 226-240. doi: 10.1007/s10461-013-0675-x

Campbell, D. T., Stanley, J. C. (1963). Experimental and quasi-experimental studies design for research. Belmont, CA: Wadsworth Cengage Learning.

Castro, R., Orozco, E., Eroza, E., Manca, M., Hernandez, J., Aggleton, P. (1998). AIDS related illness trajectories in Mexico: Findings from a qualitative study in two marginalized communities. *AIDS Care, 10*(5), 583-598.

Center for Disease Control and Prevention. (2010). Gay and bisexual men's health: stigma and discrimination. Retrieved from http://www.cdc.gov/msmhealth/stigma-and-discrimination.htm

Center for Disease Control and Prevention. (2011). National HIV Behavioral Surveillance System: Eligibility screener. Retrieved from http://www.cdc.gov/hiv/pdf/NHBS_Round3_OMBApprovedQuestionnaire-508remediated.pdf

Center for Disease Control and Prevention. (2012). Terms, definitions, and calculations used in CDC HIV surveillance publications. Retrieved from http://www.cdc.gov/hiv/pdf/prevention_ongoing_surveillance_terms.pdf

Center for Disease Control and Prevention. (2013a). HIV and AIDS among gay and

bisexual men. Retrieved from http://www.cdc.gov/nchhstp/newsroom/docs/CDC-

MSM-508.pdf

Center for Disease Control and Prevention. (2013b). Update to Interim Guidance for Pre-

exposure Prophylaxis (PrEP) for the Prevention of HIV Infection: PrEP for

injecting drug users. *Morbidity and Mortality Weekly Report, 62*(23), 463-465.

Center for Disease Control and Prevention. (2013c). HIV among African Americans.

Retrieved from http://www.cdc.gov/hiv/topics/aa/

Center for Disease Control and Prevention. (2013d). HIV among gay, bisexual, and other

men who have sex with men. Retrieved from

http://www.cdc.gov/hiv/risk/gender/msm/facts/index.html

Center for Disease Control and prevention. (2013e). Pre-exposure prophylaxis (PrEP):

Questions and answers. Retrieved from

http://www.cdc.gov/hiv/prevention/research/prep/

Center for Disease Control and prevention. (2013f). Preexposure prophylaxis (PrEP):

Questions and answers. Retrieved from

http://www.cdc.gov/hiv/prevention/research/prep/

Center for Disease Control and Prevention. (2013g). Behavioral risk factor surveillance

system. Retrieved from http://www.cdc.gov/brfss/about/brfss_faq.htm#11

Center for Disease Control and Prevention. (2014a). About HIV/AIDS. Retrieved from

http://www.cdc.gov/hiv/basics/whatishiv.html

Center for Disease Control and Prevention. (2014b). HIV among African American gay and bisexual men. Retrieved from http://www.cdc.gov/hiv/risk/racialethnic/bmsm/facts/

Chemicals, F., Recipes, H. E., Dish, B. M., Dish, P. M., Dish, S. M., Dish, P. M., ... & Calbeans, E. (2011). HIV Surveillance---United States, 1981--2008. *Morbidity and Mortality Weekly Report (MMWR)*, *60*(21), 689-693

Cohall, A., Nye, A., Moon-Howard, J., Kukafka, R., Dye, B., Vaughan, R., & Northridge, M. (2011). Computer use, internet access, and online health searching among Harlem adults. *American Journal of Health Promotion*, *25*(5), 325-333. doi:10.4278/ajhp.090325-QUAN-121

Choopanya, K., Martin, M., Suntharasamai, P., Sangkum, U., Mock, P. A. (2013). Antiretroviral prophylaxis for HIV infection in injecting drug users in Bangkok, Thailand (the Bangkok Tenofovir Study): a randomised, double-blind, placebo-controlled phase 3 trial. *Lancet 381*, 2083–2090. doi: 10.1016/s0140-6736(13)61127-7

Courtenay-Quirk, C., Pals, S. L., Colfax, G., McKirnan, D., Gooden, L., Eroglu, D. (2008). Factors associated with sexual risk behavior among persons living with HIV: Gender and sexual identity group differences. *AIDS Behavior*. 2008; 12(5):685–94. doi:10.1007/s10461-007-9259-y.

Daddario, D. K. (2007). A review of the use of the health belief model for weight management. *Medsurg Nursing*, *16*(6), 363-6.

De Man, J., Colebunders, R., Florence, E., Laga, M., Kenyon, C. (2013). What is the

place of pre-exposure prophylaxis in HIV prevention? *AIDS Review 15*, 102–111.

Dentato, M. P. (2012). The minority stress perspective. Retrieved from

http://www.apa.org/pi/aids/resources/exchange/2012/04/minority-stress.aspx

Diaz, V. (2012). Encouraging participation of minorities in research studies. Retrieved

from http://www.annfammed.org/content/10/4/372.full

Dirks, H., Esser, S., Borgmann, R., Wolter, M., Fischer, E., Potthoff, A., & ...

Scherbaum, N. (2012). Substance use and sexual risk behaviour among HIV-

positive men who have sex with men in specialized out-patient clinics. *HIV

Medicine, 13*(9), 533-540. doi:10.1111/j.1468-1293.2012.01005.x

Dorell, C., Sutton, M., Oster, A., Hardnett, F., Thomas, P., Gaul, Z., & ... Heffelfinger, J.

(2011). Missed opportunities for HIV testing in health care settings among young

African American men who have sex with men: implications for the HIV

epidemic. *AIDS Patient Care and sexually Transmitted Diseases, 25*(11), 657-

664. doi:10.1089/apc.2011.0203

Drezner, M., & Golden, R. (2012). Transforming the research environment and culture

for the betterment of health in Wisconsin. *WMJ: Official Publication of the State

Medical Society of Wisconsin, 111*(2), 89-90.

Ehlers, V., Zuyderduin, A., Oosthuizen, M. (2001). The well-being of gays, lesbians and

bisexuals in Botswana. *Journal of Advanced Nursing*, 35(6), 848-856.

Elst, E., Mbogua, J., Operario, D., Mutua, G., Kuo, C., Mugo, P., & ... Sanders, E.
(2013). High acceptability of HIV preexposure prophylaxis but Challenges in
Adherence and Use: Qualitative insights from a phase I trial of intermittent and
daily PrEP in at-risk populations in Kenya. *AIDS & Behavior, 17*(6), 2162-2172.
doi: 10.1007/s10461-012-0317-8

Ennis, C. A. (1999). A theoretical Framework: The central piece of a research plan.
*Journal of Teaching in physical Education, 18*, 129-140

Family Health International (n.d.). *Qualitative research data: A data collector's field
guide*. Retrieved from
http://www.ccs.neu.edu/course/is4800sp12/resources/qualmethods.pdf

Feldman, M. (2010). A critical literature review to identify possible causes of higher rates
of HIV infection among young black and Latino men who have sex with men.
*Journal of the National Medical Association, 102*(12), 1206-1221.

Francis, A., Mialon, H. (2010). Tolerance and HIV. *Journal of Health Economics, 29*(2),
250-267.

Frankfort-Nachmias, C., & Nachmias, D. (2008). *Research methods in the social
sciences*. New York, NY: Worth Publishers.

Freimuth, V. S., & Hovick, S. R. (2012). Cognitive and emotional health risk
perceptions among people living in poverty. *Journal of Health Communication,
17*(3), 303-318.

Galarneau, C. (2010). Blood donation, deferral, and discrimination: FDA donor deferral policy for men who have sex with men. *American Journal of Bioethics*, *10*(2), 29-39. doi:10.1080/15265160903487619

García-Lerma, J., Otten, R., Qari, S., Jackson, E., Cong, M., Masciotra, S., & ... Heneine, W. (2008). Prevention of rectal SHIV transmission in macaques by daily or intermittent prophylaxis with emtricitabine and tenofovir. *Plos Medicine*, *5*(2), e28. doi:10.1371/journal.pmed.0050028

Gates, G. J. (2006). Same sex couples and the gay, lesbian, bisexual population: New estimates from the American community survey. *The Williams Institute on Sexual Orientation Law and Public Policy, UCLA School of Law*. Retrieved from http://williamsinstitute.law.ucla.edu/wp-content/uploads/Gates-Same-Sex-Couples-GLB-Pop-ACS-Oct-2006.pdf

Gerend, M., & Shepherd, J. (2012). Predicting human papillomavirus vaccine uptake in young adult women: comparing the health belief model and theory of planned behavior. *Annals of Behavioral Medicine: A Publication of the Society of Behavioral Medicine*, *44*(2), 171-180.

Glanz, K., Rimer, B. K. & Lewis, F. M. (2002). *Health behavior and health education: Theory, research and practice*. San Francisco: Wiley & Sons

Golub, S. A., Gamarel, K. E., Rendina, H., Surace, A., & Lelutiu-Weinberger, C. L. (2013). From efficacy to effectiveness: Facilitators and barriers to PrEP acceptability and motivations for adherence among MSM and transgender women in New York City. *AIDS Patient Care & Sexually Transmitted Diseases, 27*(4), 248-254. doi:10.1089/apc.2012.0419

Granello, D. H., Wheaton, J. (2004). Online data collection: Strategies for research. *Journal of Counseling and Development, 8*(4), P. 387. Retrieved from http://imet.csus.edu/imet9/250/docs/Online_Survey.pdf

Grant, R. M., Lama, J. R., Anderson, P. L., McMahan, V., & Liu, A. Y. (2010). Preexposure chemoprophylaxis for HIV prevention in men who have sex with men. *New England Journal of Medicine 363*, 2587–2599. doi: 10.1056/nejmoa1011205

Greenlaw, C., & Brown-Welty, S. (2009). A comparison of web-based and paper-based survey methods: testing assumptions of survey mode and response cost. *Evaluation Review, 33*(5), 464-480. doi: 10.1177/0193841X09340214

Green, S. B., & Salkind, N. J. (2012). *Using SPSS for Windows and Macintosh: Analyzing and understanding data.* Boston, MA: Pearson/Prentice Hall.

Hall, H., Byers, R., Ling, Q., & Espinoza, L. (2007). Racial/ethnic and age disparities in HIV prevalence and disease progression among men who have sex with men in the United States. *American Journal of Public Health, 97*(6), 1060-1066. doi:10.2105/AJPH.2006.087551

Hampton, M., Halkitis, P., Storholm, E., Kupprat, S., Siconolfi, D., Jones, D., & ... McCree, D. (2013). Sexual risk taking in relation to sexual identification, age, and education in a diverse sample of African American men who have sex with men (MSM) in New York City. *AIDS and Behavior*, *17*(3), 931-938.

Hosek, S. G. (2013). HIV pre-exposure prophylaxis diffusion and implementation issues in nonclinical settings. *American Journal of Preventive Medicine 44*, S129–132. doi: 10.1016/j.amepre.2012.09.032

Hunter, L. (2012). Challenging the reported disadvantages of e-questionnaires and addressing methodological issues of online data collection. *Nurse Researcher*, *20*(1), 11-20.

Hounton, S., Carabin, H., & Henderson, N. (2005). Towards an understanding of barriers to condom use in rural Benin using the Health Belief Model: a cross sectional survey. *BMC Public Health*, *58*

Hurt, C.B., Eron, J.J., Cohen, M.S. (2011). Preexposure prophylaxis and antiretroviral resistance: HIV prevention at a cost? Clinical Infectious Diseases 53, 1265–1270. doi: 10.1093/cid/cir684

Jacobson, S. (2011). HIV/AIDS interventions in an aging U.S. population. *Health & Social Work*, *36*(2), 149-156.

Janz, N., & Becker, M. (1984). The Health Belief Model: A decade later. *Health Education Quarterly*, *11*(1), 1-47.

Juusola, J. L., Brandeau, M.L., Owens, D.K., & Bendavid, E. (2012). The cost-effectiveness of preexposure prophylaxis for HIV prevention in the United States in men who have sex with men. *Annals of Internal Medicine 156*, 541–550. doi: 10.7326/0003-4819-156-8-201204170-00004

Karris, M., Beekmann, S., Mehta, S., Anderson, C., & Polgreen, P. (2013). Are we prepped for PrEP? Provider opinions on the real-world use of PrEP in the U.S. and Canada. *Clinical Infectious Diseases: An Official Publication of the Infectious Diseases Society of America,*

Kilmer, J.R., Hunt, S.B., Lee, C.M., & Neighbors, C. (2007). Marijuana use, risk perception, and consequences: Is perceived risk congruent with reality? *Addictive Behaviors, 32,* 3026–3033.

Konstan, J. A., Rosser, B. R. S., Ross, M. W., Stanton, J., & Edwards, W. M. *(2005).* The story of subject naught: A cautionary but optimistic tale of Internet survey research. *Journal of Computer-Mediated Communication, 10* (2), article 11. Retrieved from *http://jcmc.indiana.edu/vol10/issue2/konstan.html.*

Kooyman, L. E. (2008). Predictors of high risk sexual behavior among gay men and men who have sex with men. *Journal of LGBT, 2*(4), 285-307

Leppin, A., & Aro, A. R. (2009). Risk perceptions related to SARS and avian influenza: Theoretical foundations of current empirical research. *International Journal of Behavioral Medicine, 16,* 7–29.

MacKellar, D., Gallagher, K., Finlayson, T., Sanchez, T., Lansky, A., & Sullivan, P. (2007). Surveillance of HIV risk and prevention behaviors of men who have sex with men--a national application of venue-based, time-space sampling. *Public Health Reports (Washington, D.C.: 1974), 122 Suppl* 139-47.

Maia, M. (2010). Rejection of the preventive discussion and at risk sexual behavior: a qualitative study among gay men in Portugal. *Sante Publique (Vandoeuvre-LesNancy, France), 22*(6), 657-664.

Marcus, J., Glidden, D., Mayer, K., Liu, A., Buchbinder, S., Amico, K., & ... Grant, R. (2013). No Evidence of Sexual Risk Compensation in the iPrEx Trial of Daily Oral HIV Preexposure Prophylaxis. *Plos One, 8*(12), e81997. doi:10.1371/journal.pone.0081997

McKirnan, D., Du Bois, S., Alvy, L., & Jones, K. (2013). Health care access and health behaviors among men who have sex with men: the cost of health disparities. *Health Education & Behavior: The Official Publication of the Society for Public Health Education, 40*(1), 32-41. doi: 10.1177/1090198111436340

Mehta, P., Sharma, M., & Lee, R. C. (2013). Designing and Evaluating a Health Belief Model-Based Intervention to Increase Intent of HPV Vaccination among College Males. *International Quarterly of Community Health Education, 34*(1), 101-117. doi:10.2190/IQ.34.1.h

Mevissen, F. F., Ruiter, R. C., Meertens, R. M., & Schaalma, H. P. (2010). The effects of scenario-based risk information on perceptions of susceptibility to Chlamydia and HIV. *Psychology & Health, 25*(10), 1161-1174

Meyer, I. H. (1995). Minority stress and mental health. Retrieved from

http://cpmcnet.columbia.edu/dept/healthandsociety/events/ms/year4/pdf/sh_Meye

r%20IH.pdf

Millett, G., Peterson, J., Flores, S., Hart, T., Jeffries, W., Wilson, P., & ... Remis, R.

(2012). Comparisons of disparities and risks of HIV infection in black and other

men who have sex with men in Canada, UK, and USA: a meta-analysis. *Lancet*,

*380*(9839), 341-348. Doi: 10.1016/S0140-6736(12)60899-X

Molina, J., Pintado, C., Gatey, C., Ponscarme, D., Charbonneau, P., Loze, B., & ...

Delaugerre, C. (2013). Challenges and opportunities for oral preexposure

prophylaxis in the prevention of HIV infection: where are we in Europe? *BMC

Medicine*, *11*186. Doi: 10.1186/1741-7015-11-186

Montanaro, E. A., & Bryan, A. D. (2013). Comparing theory-based condom

interventions: Health belief model versus theory of planned behavior. *Health

Psychology*, doi: 10.1037/a0033969

Murray, J., Kelleher, A., & Cooper, D. (2011). Timing of the components of the HIV life

cycle in productively infected CD4+ T cells in a population of HIV-infected

individuals. *Journal of Virology*, *85*(20), 10798-10805. doi:10.1128/JVI.05095-11

Myers, H., Satz, P., Miller, B., Bing, E., Evang, G., Richardson, M., Mena, I. (1997). The

African American health project: Study overview and select findings on high risk

behaviors and psychiatric disorders in African American men. *Ethnicity & health*,

2(3), 183-196.

New York City Department of Health. (2011). HIV risk and prevalence among NYC men

who have sex with men. Retrieved from

http://www.nyc.gov/html/doh/downloads/pdf/dires/nyc-msm-hiv-risk-feb6-2012-

grand-rounds.pdf

Norton, W. E., Larson, R. S., Dearing, J.W. (2013). Primary care and public health

partnerships for implementing pre-exposure prophylaxis. *American Journal of*

*Preventive Medicine 44*, S77–79. doi: 10.1016/j.amepre.2012.09.037

Oleckno, W. A. (2002). *Essential epidemiology: Principles and applications*. Prospect

Heights, Ill: Waveland.

Olmstead, T., Sindelar, J. (2004). To what extent are key services offered in treatment

programs for special population? *Journal of Substance Abuse Treatment, 27*(1), 9-

15.

Osmond, D., Pollack, L., Paul, J., & Catania, J. (2007). Changes in prevalence of HIV

infection and sexual risk behavior in men who have sex with men in San

Francisco: 1997 2002. *American Journal of Public Health, 97*(9), 1677-1683.

doi:10.2105/AJPH.2005.062851

Oster, A., Russell, K., Wiegand, R., Valverde, E., Forrest, D., Cribbin, M., & ... Paz-

Bailey, G. (2013). HIV infection and testing among Latino men who have sex

with men in the United States: the role of location of birth and other social

determinants. *Plos One, 8*(9), e73779. doi:10.1371/journal.pone.0073779

Outlaw, A. Y., Phillips, G., Hightow-Weidman, L. B., Fields, S. D., Hidalgo, J., Halpern-Felsher, B., & Study Group, ,. (2011). Age of MSM Sexual Debut and Risk Factors: Results from a Multisite Study of Racial/Ethnic Minority YMSM Living with HIV. *AIDS Patient Care & Sexually Transmitted Diseases, 25,* S23-9. doi:10.1089/apc.2011.9879

Paltiel, A., Freedberg, K., Scott, C., Schackman, B., Losina, E., Wang, B., & ... Walensky, R. (2009). HIV preexposure prophylaxis in the United States: Impacts of lifetime infection risk, clinical outcomes, and cost-effectiveness. Clinical Infectious Disease: *Clinical Infectious Diseases: An Official Publication Of The Infectious Diseases Society Of America, 48*(6), 806-815. doi: 10.1086/597095

Raymond, H., & McFarland, W. (2009). Racial mixing and HIV risk among men who have sex with men. *AIDS and Behavior, 13*(4), 630-637. doi: 10.1007/s10461-009-9574-6

Raymond, H., Chen, Y., Stall, R., & McFarland, W. (2011). Adolescent experiences of discrimination, harassment, connectedness to community and comfort with sexual orientation reported by adult men who have sex with men as a predictor of adult HIV status. *AIDS and Behavior, 15*(3), 550-556. doi: 10.1007/s10461-009-9634-y

Reid, A. E., & Aiken, L. S. (2011). Integration of five health behavior models: Common strengths and unique contributions to understanding condom use. *Psychology & Health, 26*(11), 1499-1520. doi:10.1080/08870446.2011.572259

Rosenberger, J. G., Reece, M., Schick, V., Herbenick, D., Novak, D. S., Van Der Pol, B.,

    Fortenberry, J. D. (2012). Condom use during most recent anal intercourse event

    among a U. S. sample of men who have sex with men. Retrieved from

    http://www.ncbi.nlm.nih.gov/pubmed/22353190

Rueda, S., Raboud, J., Rourke, S., Bekele, T., Bayoumi, A., Lavis, J., & ... Mustard, C.

    (2012). Influence of employment and job security on physical and mental health

    in adults living with HIV: cross-sectional analysis. *Open Medicine: A Peer-*

    *Reviewed, Independent, Open-Access Journal, 6*(4), e118-e126.

Saberi, P., Gamarel, K., Neilands, T., Comfort, M., Sheon, N., Darbes, L., & Johnson, M.

    (2012). Ambiguity, ambivalence, and apprehensions of taking HIV-1 pre-

    exposure prophylaxis among male couples in San Francisco: a mixed methods

    study. *Plos One, 7*(11), e50061. doi:10.1371/journal.pone.0050061

San Francisco AIDS Foundation. (2011). HIV/AIDS facts. Retrieved from

    http://greaterthanone.org/about/hivaids-facts.html

Semp, D., Madgeskind, S. (2000). Gay practices for harm reduction: Inviting lesbians,

    gay men and takataapui to be part of alcohol and drug harm reduction. Journal of

    Substance Use, *5*(2), 92-98.

Schneider, J., Dandona, R., Pasupneti, S., Lakshmi, V., Liao, C., Yeldandi, V., & Mayer,

    K. (2010). Initial commitment to pre-exposure prophylaxis and circumcision for

    HIV prevention amongst Indian truck drivers. *Plos One, 5*(7), e11922.

    doi:10.1371/journal.pone.0011922

Smit, P.J., Brady, M., Carter, M., Fernandes, R., & Lamore, L. (2012). HIV-related
stigma within communities of gay men: a literature review.  AIDS Care 24: 405–
412. doi:10.1080/09540121.2011.613910

Smith, D., Grant, R., Weidle, P., Lansky, A., Mermin, J., & Fenton, K. (2011). Interim
guidance: preexposure prophylaxis for the prevention of HIV infection in men
who have sex with men. *MMWR Morb Mortal Wkly Rep*, 60(3), 65-8.

Sowell, R. (2005). What does sport have to do with AIDS? *JANAC: Journal of the
Association of Nurses in AIDS Care, 16*(4), 1-2.

Statistical Solutions. (2014). Assumptions of logistic regression. Retrieved from
https://www.statisticssolutions.com/assumptions-of-logistic-regression/

Subbarao, S., Otten, R., Ramos, A., Kim, C., Jackson, E., Monsour, M., & ... Folks, T.
(2006). Chemoprophylaxis with tenofovir disoproxil fumarate provided partial
protection against infection with simian human immunodeficiency virus in
macaques given multiple virus challenges. *The Journal of Infectious Diseases,
194*(7), 904-911.

Supervie, V., García-Lerma, J. G., Heneine, W., & Blower, S. (2010). HIV, transmitted
drug resistance, and the paradox of preexposure prophylaxis. *PNAS 107 (27)
12381-12386*

Survey Monkey. (2014). What is the enhanced security option (SSL encryption)?
Retrieved from http://help.surveymonkey.com/articles/en_US/kb/What-is-the-
enhanced-security-option-SSL-encryption

Tellalian, D., Maznavi, K., Bredeek, U., & Hardy, W. (2013). Pre-Exposure Prophylaxis (PrEP) for HIV Infection: Results of a Survey of HIV Healthcare Providers Evaluating Their Knowledge, Attitudes, and Prescribing Practices. *AIDS Patient Care & Sexually Transmitted Diseases, 27*(10), 553-559. doi:10.1089/apc.2013.0173

University of Massachusetts. (2013). Online survey consent template. Retrieved from http://www.umass.edu/research/forms/online-survey-consent-template

University of North Carolina. (2010). Determining the sample size. Retrieved from http://www.unc.edu/~rls/s151-2010/class23.pdf

Vives, A., Ferreccio, C., & Marshall, G. (2009). [A comparison of two methods to adjust for non-response bias: field substitution and weighting non-response adjustments based on response propensity]. *Gaceta Sanitaria / S.E.S.P.A.S, 23*(4), 266-271. doi:10.1016/j.gaceta.2009.01.006

Vosbergen, S., Mahieu, G., Laan, E., Kraaijenhagen, R., Jaspers, M., & Peek, N. (2014). Evaluating a web-based health risk assessment with tailored feedback: what does an expert focus group yield compared to a web-based end-user survey? *Journal of Medical Internet Research, 16*(1), e1. doi:10.2196/jmir.2517

Vosburgh, H., Mansergh, G., Sullivan, P., & Purcell, D. (2012). A review of the literature on event-level substance use and sexual risk behavior among men who have sex with men. *AIDS and Behavior, 16*(6), 1394-1410. Doi: 10.1007/s10461-011-0131-8

Wade Taylor, S., Mayer, K., Elsesser, S., Mimiaga, M., O'Cleirigh, C., & Safren, S. (2013). Optimizing Content for Preexposure Prophylaxis (PrEP) Counseling for Men Who Have Sex with Men: Perspectives of PrEP Users and High-Risk PrEP Naïve Men. *AIDS and Behavior,*

Warren, J., Fernández, M., Harper, G., Hidalgo, M., Jamil, O., & Torres, R. (2008). Predictors of unprotected sex among young sexually active African American, Hispanic, and White MSM: the importance of ethnicity and culture. *AIDS and Behavior, 12*(3), 459-468.

Woolf-King, S., Rice, T., Truong, H., Woods, W., Jerome, R., & Carrico, A. (2013). Substance use and HIV risk behavior among men who have sex with men: the role of sexual compulsivity. *Journal of Urban Health: Bulletin of the New York Academy of Medicine, 90*(5), 948-952. doi: 10.1007/s11524-013-9820-0

World Health Organization (2012). Guidance on preexposure oral prophylaxis (PrEP) for serodiscordant couples, men and transgender women who have sex with men at high risk of HIV: recommendations for use in the context of demonstration projects. Geneva: WHO.

World Health Organization (2014a). Antiretroviral therapy. Retrieved from http://www.who.int/topics/antiretroviral_therapy/en/

Wright, K. B. (2006). Researching internet-based populations: Advantages and disadvantages of online survey research, online questionnaire authoring software packages, and web survey services. *Journal of Computer-Mediated Communication, Vol. 10 (3), 00, DOI: 10.1111/j.1083-6101.2005.tb00259.x*

Xiao, Z., Li, X., Lin, D., Jiang, S., Liu, Y., & Li, S. (2013). Sexual communication, safer sex self-efficacy, and condom use among young Chinese migrants in Beijing, China. *AIDS Education and Prevention: Official Publication of the International Society for AIDS Education, 25*(6), 480-494. doi:10.1521/aeap.2013.25.6.480

Zablotska, I. B., Prestage, G., de Wit, J., Grulich, A. E., Mao, L., Holt, M. (2013). Informal use of antiretrovirals for prophylaxis of HIV infection among gay men in Australia. *Journal of Acquired Immune Defficiency Syndromes, 62*(3), 334-8